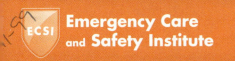

ECSI **Emergency Care and Safety Institute**

Sports First Aid and Injury Prevention

Ronald P. Pfeiffer, EdD, ATC
Medical Writer

Alton Thygerson, EdD, EMT, FAWM
Medical Writer

Nicholas F. Palmieri, DC, MPH, EMT-P
Medical Writer

Benjamin Gulli, MD
Medical Editor

Eric W. Ossman, MD, FACEP
Medical Editor

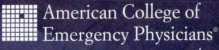

American College of
Emergency Physicians®

ADVANCING EMERGENCY CARE

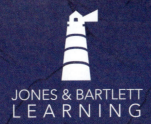

JONES & BARTLETT
LEARNING

Jones & Bartlett Learning

World Headquarters
5 Wall Street
Burlington, MA 01803
info@jblearning.com
www.ECSInstitute.org

Jones & Bartlett Learning books and products are available through most bookstores and online booksellers. To contact Jones & Bartlett Learning directly, call 800-832-0034, fax 978-443-8000, or visit our website www.jblearning.com.

Substantial discounts on bulk quantities of Jones & Bartlett Learning publications are available to corporations, professional associations, and other qualified organizations. For details and specific discount information, contact the special sales department at Jones & Bartlett Learning via the above contact information or send an email to special-sales@jblearning.com.

Production Credits
Chief Executive Officer: Clayton E. Jones
Chief Operating Officer: Donald W. Jones, Jr.
President, Higher Education and Professional Publishing:
  Robert W. Holland, Jr.
V.P., Sales and Marketing: William J. Kane
V.P., Production and Design: Anne Spencer
V.P., Manufacturing and Inventory Control: Therese Connell
Publisher, Public Safety Group: Kimberly Brophy
Acquisitions Editor: Christine Emerton

Associate Editor: Amanda Brandt
Production Manager: Jenny L. Corriveau
Associate Photo Researcher: Christine McKeen
Director of Marketing: Alisha Weisman
Interior Design: Anne Spencer
Cover Design: Kristin E. Ohlin
Cover Image: © Corbis/age fotostock
Composition: NK Graphics
Text Printing and Binding: Courier Companies
Cover Printing: Courier Companies

The first aid, CPR, and AED procedures in this book are based on the most current recommendations of responsible medical sources. The American Academy of Orthopaedic Surgeons and the Publisher, however, make no guarantee as to, and assume no responsibility for, the correctness, sufficiency, or completeness of such information or recommendations. Other or additional safety measures may be required under particular circumstances.

Some images in this book feature models. These models do not necessarily endorse, represent, or participate in the activities represented in the images.

Reviewed by the American College of Emergency Physicians

The American College of Emergency Physicians (ACEP) makes every effort to ensure that its product and program reviewers are knowledgeable content experts and recognized authorities in their fields. Readers are nevertheless advised that the statements and opinions expressed in this publication are provided as guidelines and should not be construed as College policy unless specifically referred to as such. The College disclaims any liability or responsibility for the consequences of any actions taken in reliance on those statements or opinions. The materials contained herein are not intended to establish policy, procedure, or a standard of care. To contact ACEP write to: PO Box 619911, Dallas, TX 75261-9911; call toll-free 800-798-1822, touch 6, or 972-550-0911.

ISBN: 978-1-4496-9520-0

Library of Congress Catologing-in-Publication Data

Pfeiffer, Ronald P.
  Sports first aid and injury prevention / Ronald P. Pfeiffer, Alton Thygerson, Nicholas F. Palmieri ; American Academy of Orthopaedic Surgeons.
      p. cm.
  Includes index.
  ISBN-13: 978-0-7637-5556-0 (pbk.)
  ISBN-10: 0-7637-5556-7 (pbk.)
  1. Sports injuries—Prevention. 2. Sports medicine. 3. Wounds and injuries—Prevention. 4. First aid in illness and injury. I. Thygerson, Alton L. II. Palmieri, Nicholas F. III. Title.
  RD97.P4814 2008
  617.1'027—dc22
                              2008006556
6048

Additional photographic and illustration credits appear on page 110, which constitutes a continuation of the copyright page.

Printed in the United States of America
16 15 14 13 12   10 9 8 7 6 5 4

contents

Chapter 1 Background Information 2

Why Train the Coach? 2
What Is Sports First Aid? 3
Sports First Aid and the Law 3
Sports First-Aid Kit 4
General Principles of Sports First Aid 4
   RICE 4
   Heat and Cold 7
Special Considerations 7
   Training and Conditioning for Youth Athletes 7
   Repetitive Stress/Overuse Injuries in Youth Athletes . . . 8
   Hydration 8
   Concussion 8
   Gender Differences 9
   Spinal Injury 9
   Drug and Alcohol Use and Abuse in Athletes 9

Chapter 2 Recognizing a Sick or Injured Athlete 10

Introduction 10
Approaching the Sick or Injured Athlete 11
Victim Assessment: Finding the Problem 12
   Initial Check 12
   Head-to-Toe Survey 12
   SAMPLE History 19
   Modifying the Assessment for Athletes 19
Getting Help 20
The Decision to Return to Play 21

Chapter 3 Caring for Sports-Related Illnesses 23

Introduction 23
Allergic Reactions 23
Choking 25
Diabetic Emergencies 25
Drug Overdose and Poisoning 25
Environmental Emergencies 26
   Cold-Related Emergencies 26
   Heat-Related Emergencies 27

Fainting 27
Heart (Cardiac) Problems 28
Hyperventilation Syndrome 28
Motionless Athlete 28
Seizures 29
Shortness of Breath (Asthma and
   Other Breathing Problems) 29
Unresponsiveness 30
Vomiting 30

Chapter 4 Caring for Sports-Related Injuries 31

Bites and Stings 31
Bleeding and Wounds 32
   Wounds that Need Suturing 33
Blisters 34
Burns 34
Contusions 36
Dislocations 36
Drowning 36
Fractures 37
   Applying a Splint 37
Sprains 38
Strains 39
Common Injuries by Region 39
   Head and Face Injuries 39
   Spine Injuries 43
   Chest Injuries 44
   Upper Extremity Injuries 45
   Lower Extremity Injuries 54

Chapter 5 Phases of Injury: The Injury Prevention Model 59

Introduction 59
The Preinjury Phase 60
   The Athlete 60
   The Environment 61
   The Rules of the Game 61
   The Officials and Coaches 61
   The Medical Team 61
   Emergency Action Plan 62

The Injury Phase 62
The Postinjury Phase 63
    Immediately Following an Injury 63
    Between the Injury and Release 63
    Before Return to Play 64
Summary of the Injury Prevention Model 64

Chapter 6   Preventing Sports-Related Injuries and Illnesses   65

Introduction 65
Contact/Collision Sports 67
    Basketball 67
    Football 68
    Ice Hockey 69
    Lacrosse 70
    Martial Arts 71
    Roller Hockey 71
    Soccer 72
    Wrestling 73
Limited Contact Sports 74
    Baseball/Softball 74
    Cheerleading 75
    Field Events 76
    Gymnastics 77
    Skiing (Alpine) 78
    Volleyball 78
Noncontact Sports 79
    Swimming 79
    Tennis 80
    Track 81
    Weight Lifting and Weight Training 81

Chapter 7   CPR and AED   84

Heart Attack and Cardiac Arrest 84
Chain of Survival 85
How the Heart Works 86
    When Normal Electrical Activity Is Interrupted 87
Care for Cardiac Arrest 87
Performing CPR 87
    Check for Responsiveness 87
    Give Chest Compressions 87
    Rescue Breaths 88
Airway Obstruction 92
    Recognizing Airway Obstruction 92
    Caring for a Person with an Airway Obstruction 92
Public Access Defibrillation 94
About AEDs 94
    Common Elements of AEDs 95
Using an AED 96
Special Considerations 98
    Water 98
    Children 98
    Medication Patches 98
    Implanted Devices 99
AED Maintenance 99
Summary 99

Appendix A: Emergency Action Plan 100

Index 101

Image Credits 110

welcome

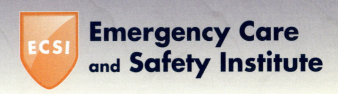

Emergency Care and Safety Institute

Welcome to the Emergency Care and Safety Institute

Welcome to the Emergency Care and Safety Institute (ECSI), brought to you by the American Academy of Orthopaedic Surgeons (AAOS) and the American College of Emergency Physicians (ACEP).

The ECSI is an educational organization created for the purpose of delivering the highest quality training to laypersons and professionals in the areas of First Aid, CPR, AED, Bloodborne Pathogens, and related safety and health fields.

Two of the most respected names in injury, illness, and emergency medical care—AAOS and ACEP—have approved the content of our training materials.

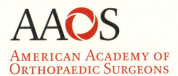

AMERICAN ACADEMY OF ORTHOPAEDIC SURGEONS

About the AAOS

The AAOS provides education and practice management services for orthopaedic surgeons and allied health professionals. The AAOS also serves as an advocate for improved patient care and informs the public about the science of orthopaedics. Founded in 1933, the not-for-profit AAOS has grown from a small organization serving less than 500 members to the world's largest medical association of musculoskeletal specialists. The AAOS now serves about 24,000 members internationally.

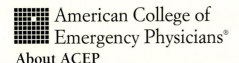

American College of Emergency Physicians®

About ACEP

ACEP was founded in 1968 and is the world's oldest and largest emergency medicine specialty organization. Today it represents more than 23,000 members and is the emergency medicine specialty society recognized as the acknowledged leader in emergency medicine.

ECSI Course Catalog

Individuals seeking training in ECSI subjects can choose from among various online and offline course offerings. The following courses are available through the ECSI:

First Aid, CPR, and AED Standard

CPR and AED

Professional Rescuer CPR

First Aid

Wilderness First Aid

Bloodborne Pathogens

First Responder

First Aid and CPR Online

First Aid Online

Adult CPR Online

Adult and Pediatric CPR Online

Professional Rescuer CPR Online

AED Online

Adult CPR and AED Online

Bloodborne Pathogens Online

The ECSI offers a wide range of textbooks, instructor and student support materials, and interactive technology, including online courses. Every ECSI textbook is the center of an integrated teaching and learning system that offers instructor, student, and technology resources to better support instructors and prepare students. The instructor supplements provide practical hands-on, time-saving tools like PowerPoint presentations, DVDs, and web-based distance learning resources. The student supplements are designed to help students retain the most important information and to assist them in preparing for exams. And, a key component to the teaching and learning systems are technology resources that provide interactive exercises and simulations to help students become great emergency responders.

Documents attesting to the ECSI's recognitions of satisfactory course completion will be issued to those who successfully meet the course objectives and criteria for passing the course. Written acknowledgement of a participant's successful course completion is provided in the form of a Course Completion Card, issued by the ECSI.

Visit www.ECSInstitute.org today!

resource preview

This textbook is designed to give athletic coaches basic first aid and injury prevention techniques to implement in both athletic practices and athletic competitions. Features that will reinforce and expand on essential information include:

Skill Drills
Provide step-by-step explanations and visual summaries of important skills for coaches.

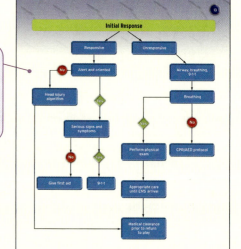

Chapter at a Glance
Guides coaches through the topics covered in that chapter.

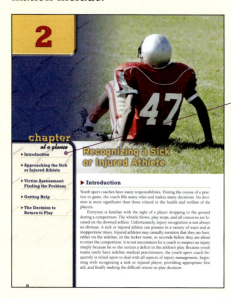

Flowcharts
Pose a central question and organize treatment options by injury or illness type.

Tip Boxes
Include valuable information about prevention and first aid related to the injuries and illnesses discussed in that section.

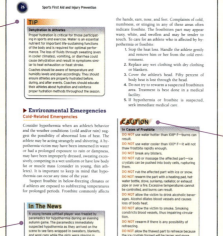

Caution Boxes
Emphasize crucial actions that coaches should or should not take while administering first aid.

In the News Boxes
Provide real-life examples of athlete illness and injuries.

Acknowledgments

Jones and Bartlett Publishers would like to thank the following individuals for their review of the manuscript:

Reviewers

Sally Becker, EMT-I
Becker Training Associates
Webster, New Hampshire

Lisa M. Cantara, MS, ATC, CSCS
Stony Brook University
Stony Brook, New York

Larry J. Cohen, BS, EMT-P
4x4 MEDIC—Emergency Care Training Services
Westminster, Maryland

Michelle Golba-Norek, RN, BSN, MICN
Raritan Bay Medical Center EMS
Perth Amboy, New Jersey

Jaime S. Greene, AAS, BA, EMT-B
Safety Associates, Inc.
West Palm Beach, Florida

Hugh W. Harling, EdD, LAT, ATC
Methodist University
Fayetteville, North Carolina

R. Scott Lauder, RN
Initial Response, Inc.
Carrollton, Virginia

Michael O. McLeieer, FF, EMT-FR
Certified National Fire Instructor
ESCAPE Fire & Safety Services, Inc.
Kalamazoo, Michigan

Angel J. Nater, BS, EMT-P
Seminole County Dept. of Public Safety
Sanford, Florida

Robb S. Rehberg, PhD, ATC, NREMT
Director of Athletic Training Education
William Paterson University
Wayne, New Jersey

Craig Spector
President 2007 National Chairperson for ECSI
EMT Instructor
CPR Heart Starters Inc Safety Training
Warrington, Pennsylvania

Rod Walters, DA, ATC
Consultant in Sports Medicine
Walters Inc.
Columbia, South Carolina

Brad D. Weilbrenner
Rockingham Regional Ambulance
Nashua, New Hampshire

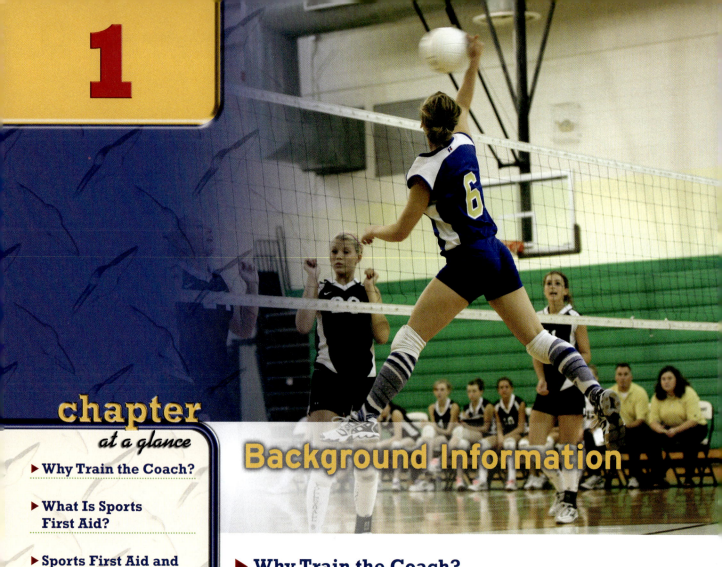

chapter
at a glance

▶ **Why Train the Coach?**

▶ **What Is Sports First Aid?**

▶ **Sports First Aid and the Law**

▶ **Sports First-Aid Kit**

▶ **General Principles of Sports First Aid**

▶ **Special Considerations**

Background Information

▶ Why Train the Coach?

The youth sport coach commonly assumes sole responsibility for recognizing and managing sudden illness or injury during a practice or game situation. Coaches frequently are forced to make return-to-play decisions and are responsible for ensuring that sick or injured athletes are followed up properly. Consider how a coach should handle the following situations:

> *You are running a hockey practice for 12-year-olds. Suddenly, during a checking drill, you notice one of your players clutching his left shoulder and wincing in pain.*
> *You are coaching a soccer team of 15-year-olds and suddenly one of your players drops to the ground. The referee runs to the injured player and calls you over. She is lying motionless on the ground. A concerned parent runs onto the field and begins shaking the girl.*
> *You are coaching a group of 8-year-old baseball players. Suddenly one of the players appears to be having difficulty breathing. The player tells you he is having an asthma attack and that he left his asthma inhaler at home. One*

of your assistant coaches, also an asthmatic, offers his asthma inhaler to the sick child.

You are a varsity high school coach preparing for a basketball game. You notice your top scorer limping into the locker room. As soon as he sees you, he hides his limp and assures you that he is OK and is ready to play.

You are running a lacrosse practice for 13-year-old boys. You are called over to check out an injured player who reportedly was "knocked out." When you initially get to him, he is awake and answering your questions but seems a little confused. He gets up and goes to the sideline. Five minutes later, he tells you he is ready to go back on the field.

These are common situations that youth sport coaches may face on a regular basis. The *Sports First Aid and Injury Prevention* program prepares the youth sport coach to deal with these and other emergency situations. At the conclusion of the course, a coach will be prepared to develop an action plan and learn when to intervene and when additional medical support is required. The coach will be trained to take immediate action to care for sick or injured athletes and to understand the proper follow-up procedures to ensure that the athlete receives appropriate medical care and that return-to-play decisions are handled appropriately (see Chapter 2).

Because many sports injuries are preventable, the coach has the added responsibility of anticipating potential injuries and implementing prevention strategies for injury control and reduction. Strategies used to minimize and control injury include appropriate conditioning programs; properly fitted equipment; and a safe playing surface, free of potential obstacles and hazards.

▶ What Is Sports First Aid?

First aid is the immediate care given to an injured or suddenly ill person. Along with first aid, *Sports First Aid and Injury Prevention* includes strategies to minimize and prevent injuries. This program will train the coach to recognize when intervention is needed and when additional medical support is required. Not only can quality first aid save someone's life,

but it can reduce disability and hospitalization and accelerate return-to-play time. The *Sports First Aid and Injury Prevention* program is not inclusive for all aspects of first aid; it is specifically for illnesses and injuries that may be encountered in athletes, particularly young athletes. Although the program prepares coaches to handle many emergencies, the program also stresses the need to implement injury prevention strategies. This program is not a substitution for medical care, and the need for follow-up care by appropriate medical providers cannot be overemphasized.

▶ Sports First Aid and the Law

"If you place the welfare of the sick or injured ahead of all other considerations, you will rarely if ever commit an unethical act in providing first aid."

Nancy Caroline, MD

Coaches, officials, and league-governing bodies must provide a safe environment for their athletes. A coach's responsibility does not end when the game or practice session has ended. The following guidelines are just a primer that can help coaches minimize risk and limit liability:

- Ensure that the physical and skill attributes of athletes are matched.
- Provide a safe environment during all team activities, including travel, practice sessions, locker room time, and team meetings.
- All practices and activities should be planned and include proper instruction and close supervision.
- Both athletes and parents must be warned of the potential risks of the sport.
- Coaches must maintain a high "index of suspicion" for potential injuries.
- When an injury occurs, it should be managed promptly and according to accepted standards of care.
- Coaches must keep adequate records and report all incidents and injuries to league-governing bodies and parents of minor athletes.

- Coaches should never place themselves in a position of risk. Never touch or examine sensitive areas and never be in a position that could be misconstrued as inappropriate. Always be sure to have someone else with you while you examine an injured athlete.
- Obtain consent before the season begins. Signed consent and emergency information data should be obtained before the first practice and kept in the coach's possession at every team event.
- Never abandon a victim. Once a coach establishes contact with a sick or injured athlete, do not leave him or her until someone with the same or higher training takes over.
- Do not be negligent. Negligence occurs when additional harm arises because someone does not follow the accepted standards of care. Many coaches refuse first-aid training because they falsely believe training will increase their liability. The duty to care for a sick or injured athlete is the responsibility of the coach. First-aid training reduces coaches' risk by preparing them to act according to currently acceptable standards. It also reduces the chance that a coach will breach his or her responsibility to act, due to lack of confidence in handling emergency situations. Negligence also can occur because the wrong care was provided and additional damage occurred. Guard against negligence by not exceeding your level of training when providing care. The *Sports First Aid and Injury Prevention* program teaches what a coach should not do as well as what actions should be taken.
- Maintain confidentiality. All coaches must keep what they know and what they see to themselves. Do not discuss incidents or an athlete's medical information with anyone other than those who must know, such as parents and other first aid or medical providers.
- Document and report each illness and injury to league administrators. Additionally, the injury log should be reviewed at the end of the season to track injury trends to implement future prevention strategies.

▶ Sports First-Aid Kit

Table 1-1 contains first-aid items for use in sports. Modify the list to meet specific needs a particular organization or group of athletes may have. Please note that this list does not include internal medications.

▶ General Principles of Sports First Aid

Use the following guidelines to ensure uniform application of first-aid principles to athletes:

- First, do no further harm.
- Take control of the situation (use bystanders to the situation's advantage).
- Try to remain calm and always reassure the victim.
- Leave the victim in the position found unless he or she is at risk of further harm.
- If the victim is lifeless, administer appropriate CPR protocols.
- Perform an initial survey, head-to-toe survey, and SAMPLE history (see Chapter 2).
- Always use common sense. Most problems encountered by coaches are not life threatening and can be guided by common sense applications.
- If a coach is ever unsure of the severity of a problem or what to do, he or she should call 9-1-1 and await the arrival of the professionals.

RICE

The mnemonic RICE can be helpful in remembering the treatment for many sports-related injuries Skill Drill 1-1 :

- R — Rest
- I — Ice
- C — Compression
- E — Elevation

Applying an elastic bandage for up to 48 hours (or as directed by a health care practitioner) after a sprain or strain reduces swelling and internal bleeding by compressing the underlying tissues. Elastic bandages come in various widths for different body parts:

Table 1-1 Sport First-Aid Kit

Item	Use
Alcohol towelettes/wipes	Clean hands and clean around wound (not inside wound)
Antibiotic ointment (example: Polysporin, Neosporin, Bacitracin, triple antibiotic ointment)	Provides best wound-healing environment Prevents skin infections associated with shallow wounds Makes nonstick dressings
Aloe vera gel (100% gel)	Soothes pain of mild sunburn and superficial frostbite
Moleskin/molefoam	Treats "hot spots" before blister formation Pads painful blisters
Irrigation syringe (20 mL or greater)	Can provide irrigation of wounds or chemical burns
Bandage strips of various sizes (example: Band-Aids)	Cover minor wounds
Sterile gauze pads (2 × 2 and 4 × 4 individually wrapped)	Cover wounds
Nonsticking pads	Cover burns, blisters, and scrapes
Self-adhering roller bandage (2-4" wide; example: Kerlix, Kling)	Secure dressings
Sterile trauma pad (5 × 9", 8 × 10")	Used as dressing for large wounds
Elastic bandage (2", 3", 4" wide; example: Ace wrap)	Provides compression to reduce swelling of joint injuries
Adhesive tape (various types available; example: athletic tape, hypoallergenic tape, waterproof tape)	Secures dressings and splints
Safety pins (2" long)	Help create sling from shirt tail or sleeve; secure dressings
Hydrocortisone cream, 1%	Soothes inflammation associated with insect bites and stings, poison ivy and oak, and other allergic skin rashes
Calamine lotion	Anti-itch and drying agent for poison ivy, poison oak, and skin rashes
Sunscreen lotion (with sun protection factor of at least 15)	Prevents sunburn, windburn
Lip balm, individual use only (with sun protection factor of 15)	Prevents sunburn, chapping of lips Soothes cold sores
Insect repellent	Repels insects
Scissors (various types are available)	Cut dressings, bandages, and clothing
Tweezers (angled tip)	Remove splinters and ticks
SAM splints (multiple sizes)	Stabilize broken bones and dislocations
Medical exam gloves	Protect against potentially infected blood and body fluids
Mouth-to-barrier device	Protects against potential infection during rescue breathing/CPR
Emergency blanket	Protects against body heat loss and weather
Small notebook/pencil	Helps in recording and sending information
Triangular bandages, cravats	Used to make slings and swaths and to stabilize injuries and splints; used as bandages
Ice packs	Provide instant access to cold to reduce swelling
Plastic bags	Used for ice application and to collect blood-soaked dressings
Emergency action plan (see Appendix A) with medical history and treatment forms attached	Lists information necessary in an emergency
Sports First Aid and Injury Prevention	Quick reference during an emergency

skill drill

1-1   RICE Procedure

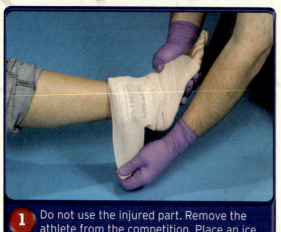

1 Do not use the injured part. Remove the athlete from the competition. Place an ice pack on the injured area. Use an elastic bandage to hold the ice pack in place for 20 minutes.

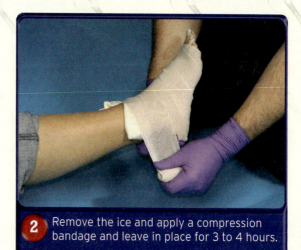

2 Remove the ice and apply a compression bandage and leave in place for 3 to 4 hours.

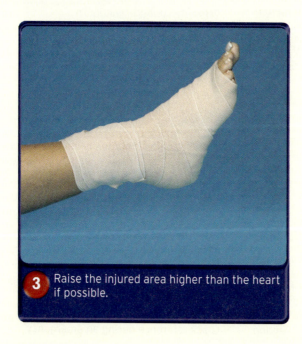

3 Raise the injured area higher than the heart if possible.

TIP

Homemade Ice Packs

- Homemade ice packs can be made using plastic freezer bags, water, and rubbing alcohol. Add three parts water and one part alcohol to a plastic freezer bag. The frozen bag will be pliable and can easily be molded to the injured area.
- For cold therapy over a fairly large area, soak a face towel in cold water, wring it out, fold it, and place it in a large, self-sealing plastic bag. Store the bag in the freezer.
- Fill a plastic bag with snow or ice cubes (keep extra plastic bags in your first-aid kit for this reason).

TIP

Ice Massage

A health care provider may recommend ice massage to an injured area. To prepare for ice massage, fill a polystyrene plastic cup with water and freeze it. When you need to perform ice massage, peel the cup to below the ice level; the remaining part of the cup forms a cold-resistant handle. Place a towel below the area being treated since the ice will melt during the application. Massage the ice over the injured area for about 5 minutes (movement is necessary to prevent skin damage).

- Two-inch width for hand, foot, and wrist
- Three-inch width for elbow, ankle, and arm
- Four-inch width for knee, leg, and shoulder

To apply an elastic bandage, start the elastic bandage several inches below the injury site and wrap in an upward overlapping (about one half to three quarters of the bandage's width) spiral starting with even moderate pressure, then gradually loosening pressure above the injured area. The bandage

CAUTION

- **DO NOT** apply an ice pack for more than 20 minutes at a time. Frostbite or nerve damage can result.
- **DO NOT** apply an ice pack to the back part of the knee. Nerve damage can occur.
- **DO NOT** apply cold if the victim has a history of circulatory disease, Raynaud's disease (spasms in the arteries of the extremities that reduce circulation), an abnormal sensitivity to cold, or if the injured part has been frostbitten previously.
- **DO NOT** stop using an ice pack too soon. A common mistake is the early use of heat, which will result in swelling and pain. Use an ice pack three to four times a day for the first 24 hours, preferably up to 48 hours. For severe injuries, using ice for up to 72 hours is recommended.

should be reapplied at least three times a day and can be removed for ice application. It should remain in place at bedtime, but can be slightly loosened.

Heat and Cold

Many people use heat devices or ice packs to speed the recovery from sports injuries, but when is the right time to use each technique? Cold can safely be applied immediately after an acute injury. Ice reduces pain, swelling, and muscle spasm immediately after injury, but its use should be discontinued after 2 or 3 days.

Heat should be used only on the advice of a medical practitioner. Heat increases circulation to an injured area, thereby reducing muscle spasm and potentially reducing pain. The use of heat too soon after an acute injury can potentially increase swelling and pain and increase healing time. Heat should not be used for at least 72 hours after an acute injury (unless directed by a health care practitioner). If symptoms of an injury persist for 72 hours, consultation with a medical practitioner is indicated. Therefore, the use of heat without direct medical consultation is not recommended.

▶ Special Considerations

Training and Conditioning for Youth Athletes

In the past, children played sports to improve or maintain their physical fitness levels while having fun. In today's world of competitive youth sports, it has become commonplace for young athletes to adopt intense training programs to maintain or enhance their physical attributes for a specific sport. Organized training programs for specific sports training exist for very young children, often believed by parents and coaches to give a competitive edge to their children. Training and conditioning for young athletes should be guided by appropriately trained individuals such as doctors, athletic trainers, and other health care providers with knowledge of the physical and psychological development of children. Conditioning programs should be age, development, and gender appropriate, with a keen eye on potentially harmful psychological and physical effects.

Repetitive Stress/Overuse Injuries in Youth Athletes

Coaches should consider the possibility of overuse injuries in their young athletes. The days of multi-sport athletes are dwindling and sport specialization is beginning at younger ages. Year-round involvement in one sport increases the possibility of overuse injuries. Coaches should be alert to the possibility of repetitive motion and overuse injuries (such as chronic tendinitis, stress fractures, and growth plate injuries) in athletes who perform repetitive tasks (for example, baseball pitchers and volleyball setters). Some youth baseball organizations have set guidelines for the number of pitches thrown by young pitchers, and other organizations may have guidelines to prevent overuse injuries. It is the responsibility of the coach to be alert and to maintain a high index of suspicion for such problems prevalent to his or her sport.

Symptoms of pain in a joint (including extremities and spine) during or soon after an activity commonly indicate trauma to the bone, muscle, tendon, or tendon–bone junction and should alert the coach to the possibility of an overuse type problem. Such symptoms could be potentially serious in young athletes and warrant medical (orthopaedic) follow-up.

Hydration

The age of the athletes, the amount of equipment worn, and the temperature and humidity levels of the environment are all important factors in determining the amount of water an individual requires. Although overhydration is possible, the practice of underhydration in youth athletes is more commonplace. Water and/or electrolyte-containing solutions are the best methods of hydrating athletes. Caution is advised in using sugar or other "performance-enhancing"–type fluid solutions for hydration purposes. It is important for coaches, especially those who deal with younger athletes, to be sure athletes are properly hydrated during practices and competitions. It may be necessary to counsel the athletes and/or their parents regarding pre- and postgame hydration requirements.

Recently there have been issues concerning the sharing of water bottles among teammates due to the possibility of spreading diseases (such as meningitis). It is strongly recommended that athletes have their own water bottles labeled with their names and numbers during each event. It is recommended that the bottles be washed with soap and water after each event.

Concussion

A *concussion* occurs when the brain is shaken violently within the skull, secondary to some outside force such as a blow to the head, neck, or upper body. Because brain activity is momentarily disrupted, symptoms such as confusion, dizziness, disorientation, memory loss, and unconsciousness may occur. Because clear findings may not show up on physical and diagnostic tests (such as CT scans and MRIs), many concussions go undiagnosed. Coaches should be alert to changes in their athletes' symptoms and mental status and offer their complete attention to those with possible concussions. Concussions are cumulative, and the severity of symptoms after three concussions increases one's risk of long-term neurologic deficits. Multiple concussions heighten the level of concern coaches and parents should have toward these injuries. Preseason (preparticipation) and postconcussion neuropsychological testing such as the ImPACT (Immediate Post-concussion Assessment and Cognitive Test) should be considered for those who participate in collision sports.

Gender Differences

Differing physical, hormonal, and psychological development in athletes may create distinctive illness and injury patterns. The coach should be familiar with rules concerning combined and gender-specific sports. The coach should be familiar with developmental issues of his or her male and female athletes and make necessary adjustments to accommodate their needs. This may include equipment modification, locker room accommodation, and an understanding of anatomic development to better understand injury patterns. Concerns regarding young female athletes compared with males include an increased risk of knee ligament injuries, reduced upper extremity strength, hormonal imbalances, and nutritional and eating disorders. The coach should be familiar with concerns of male and female athletes and seek proper counsel regarding prevention and management of such issues as well as maintaining a high index of suspicion for their existence.

Spinal Injury

With increased participation in youth sports, especially contact sports, comes the increased incidence of spinal injury. Annually, approximately 11,000 people in the United States sustain spinal cord injury. Many of these injuries result from sport participation by people younger than 35 years of age.

Spinal cord injury has profound effects on the victim's life. Not only does a victim have to deal with the physical limitations, but spinal cord injuries may result in abnormal functioning of many of the body functions. In addition, the lifelong financial consequences can be devastating. As these injuries occur suddenly, emphasis must be placed on proper conditioning, appropriate equipment, and proper education. Many sports, such as ice hockey, have formal programs such as the "heads-up" contact programs that can be presented to participants to teach proper methods of body contact.

When a spinal cord injury does occur, prompt recognition and appropriate early management can have profound effects on the outcome. Every coach needs to be aware of the potential for such injuries in his or her sport and understand the critical importance of immediate spinal immobilization procedures when such an injury occurs.

Drug and Alcohol Use and Abuse in Athletes

Coaches should be aware of prescription and illicit drug use in athletes for recreational, social, and performance enhancement uses. Athletes sometimes are pressured into the use of anabolic steroids and other performance-enhancing substances to improve sports performance without understanding the long-term risks and/or medical and legal complications that commonly accompany these substances. Illicit drugs (including designer drugs, alcohol, and marijuana) and misused prescription drugs can cause a variety of problems in young athletes. Coaches should consider the possibility of drug or alcohol use in athletes with unexplained behavior, a sudden change in performance, or other unexplained sudden illness. Coaches must support drug screening programs and drug awareness education programs in young athletes.

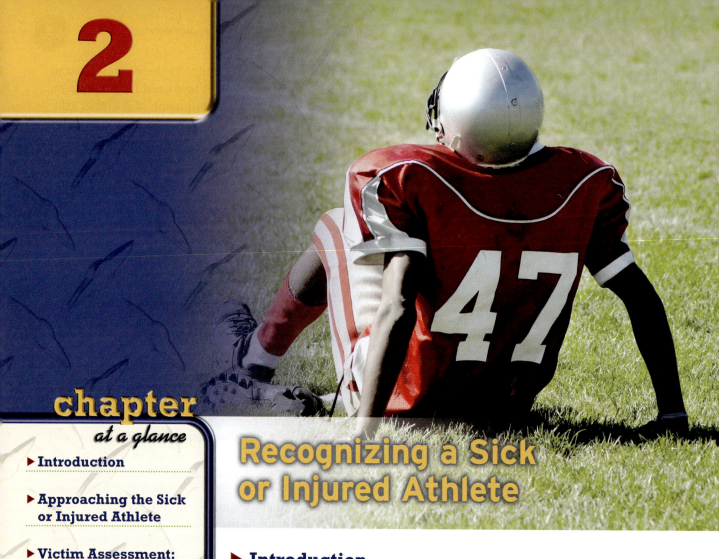

2

chapter *at a glance*

▶ **Introduction**

▶ **Approaching the Sick or Injured Athlete**

▶ **Victim Assessment: Finding the Problem**

▶ **Getting Help**

▶ **The Decision to Return to Play**

Recognizing a Sick or Injured Athlete

▶ Introduction

Youth sport coaches have many responsibilities. During the course of a practice or game, the coach fills many roles and makes many decisions. No decision is more significant than those related to the health and welfare of the players.

Everyone is familiar with the sight of a player dropping to the ground during a competition. The whistle blows, play stops, and all concerns are focused on the downed athlete. Unfortunately, injury recognition is not always so obvious. A sick or injured athlete can present in a variety of ways and at inopportune times. Injured athletes may casually mention that they are hurt, either on the sideline, in the locker room, or seconds before they are about to enter the competition. It is not uncommon for a coach to suspect an injury simply because he or she notices a deficit in the athlete's play. Because youth teams rarely have sideline medical practitioners, the youth sport coach frequently is relied upon to deal with all aspects of injury management, beginning with recognizing a sick or injured player, providing appropriate first aid, and finally making the difficult return-to-play decision.

The assessment of a situation begins as soon as the coach realizes that someone is in distress. An emergency action plan (EAP) should be activated at this time. As the coach approaches the victim, he or she should observe the playing field and query whether anyone else is injured. At the same time, the coach should begin to anticipate potentially injured areas. As an expert in that sport, the coach should understand the forces involved and common injuries experienced by athletes in that particular event. If they observed the injury, coaches can begin to speculate what injuries may have occurred. Experienced coaches can identify injuries simply by watching how the player goes down. Look for clues:

- Is this a medical problem, such as an asthma attack?
- Is this an injury?
- Is there obvious damage to any equipment?
- Are there any evident deformities, blood, or bruising?
- What are the other players saying?

It is not uncommon for youth athletes to describe boldly a bone-jarring hit or the sound of a "cracking" bone. Once the coach reaches the sick or injured athlete, a more thorough assessment can begin. Ignore for a moment the momentum of the competition. The coach should arrive at the victim's side with confidence and concern.

In The News

A soccer coach inadvertently dislocated a young athlete's finger. The coach was tending to the injured girl and stepped on her hand while turning to yell at the referee for not calling a penalty on the play.

▶ Approaching the Sick or Injured Athlete

A coach should be aware of inherent risks associated with providing first aid. It is important to ensure that they themselves are in no danger and that any additional risk of injury to the victim is minimized. In addition, the first-aid provider must take steps to protect him- or herself from any infectious disease that can be spread through blood or bodily fluid contact. As the coach approaches the injured athlete he or she must consider potential obstacles and appropriate footing and ensure complete stoppage of play.

In The News

A baseball coach was injured when he stepped on the field to tend to an injured shortstop. Play was not stopped and the coach was hit by a line drive.

Certain diseases could be transmitted by contact with an infected victim. Infectious diseases are viruses and bacteria that can be transmitted from one person to another. Although the risk of acquiring a disease while rendering first aid is low, simple measures taken as protection from blood and airborne disease can lower the risk even more. Protection begins with confirmation of the coach's own immunization status against tetanus and hepatitis B. The coach also should verify that the athletes' immunizations are current and he or she should be aware of any players that may have an infectious disease. As a coach reaches for the first-aid kit, personal protective equipment such as gloves and eye protection should be readily accessible at the top of the kit.

A coach can protect him- or herself by following these steps:

- Use gloves and consider eye protection. Gloves, barrier devices, and protective glasses should be part of the first-aid kit.
- Use a barrier device, such as a face shield or pocket mask, when providing rescue breaths.
- Wash hands with soap and water after each incident.
- Dispose of exposed items in appropriate waste disposal containers (if medical waste bags are not available, place the blood-stained items in double-sealed plastic bags until they can be disposed of properly).
- Cover any open wounds on their body with a dressing.

- Be properly immunized (tetanus and hepatitis B).
- Do not eat, drink, or touch their face while providing care.
- Clean contaminated areas and equipment with an appropriate cleaning solution. A diluted bleach solution (fresh mixture of 0.25 cup household bleach to a gallon of water) usually is sufficient.

▶ Victim Assessment: Finding the Problem

Once the coach arrives at the victim's side, he or she should identify and correct any life-threatening problems before doing anything else. If the coach deems a life-threatening or serious condition is present, he or she should summon additional help by having someone call 9-1-1 or the local emergency number immediately.

Two assessments (initial check and head-to-toe survey) and a SAMPLE history are used to ensure a complete evaluation. Most victims do not require a complete head-to-toe survey and not all parts of an assessment apply to every victim. Different problems and conditions require different approaches for identifying what is wrong. The coach likely will approach an injured victim differently than a sick victim.

Initial Check

The initial check identifies immediate life-threatening conditions and can be completed in seconds. Problems discovered during the initial check should be cared for before continuing the assessment. The coach should begin by checking the victim's level of responsiveness and for signs of life. If the victim is responsive, the coach can be assured that he or she is breathing and has a pulse. If this is the case, the coach can assess the level of responsiveness Table 2-1 and continue to the head-to-toe survey. If the victim is unresponsive, seek immediate medical care by calling 9-1-1 or the local emergency number. Check the athlete's breathing and check for life-threatening bleeding. Use of the mnemonics RAP and CABD will help to remember the sequence

Table 2-2 . The initial check may indicate a need for cardiopulmonary resuscitation (CPR) or use of an automated external defibrillator (AED). CPR and use of an AED are explained further in Chapter 7.

Head-to-Toe Survey

The head-to-toe survey attempts to locate other injuries or additional clues to a victim's condition. Unless you encounter a potentially life-threatening injury during the head-to-toe survey, do not stop to tend to injuries until the survey is completed. This ensures a complete evaluation and will minimize the risk of missing subtle problems.

The head-to-toe survey ensures that a coach evaluates the entire victim to detect anything out of the ordinary Skill Drill 2-1 . Use the mnemonic "LAF for DOTS" from head to toe to help remember the sequence and ensure a thorough assessment.

LAF is a mnemonic for "look and feel." DOTS is a mnemonic for:

Deformity—Observe for malformed or misshaped areas (compare with uninjured part).

Open wounds—Observe for bleeding.

Tenderness—Take note of sensitive or painful areas when touched.

Swelling—Observe for distended or swollen areas (compare with uninjured part).

Look and feel (LAF) for deformity, open wounds, tenderness, and swelling (DOTS).

Table 2-1 Assessing Level of Responsiveness		
	Ask the Victim	**Can Be Modified for the Athlete**
Person	What is your name?	What is the name of your team?
Place	Where are you?	What team are you playing against?
Time	What day (time) is it?	What quarter (inning, period) is it?

Initial Response

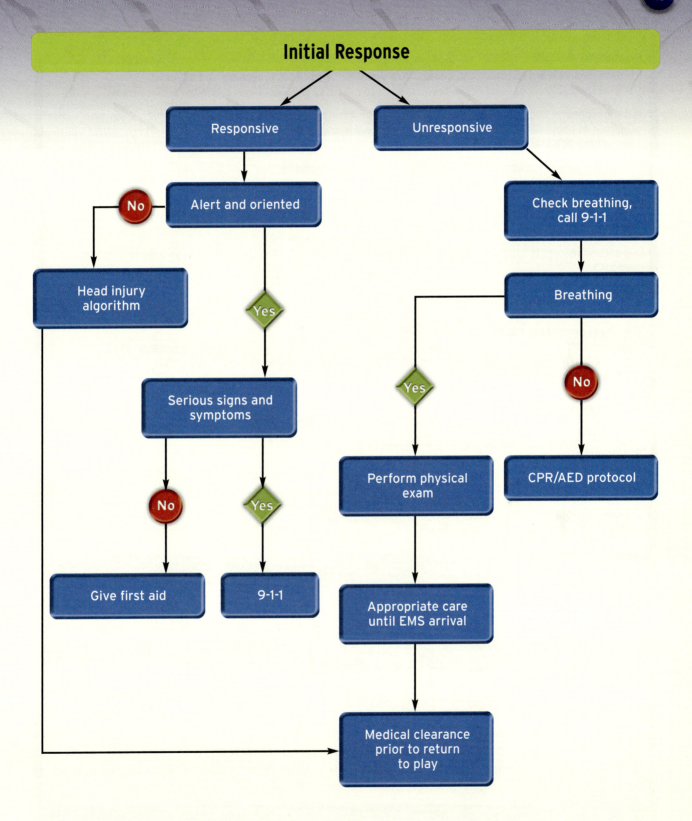

Table 2-2 Initial Check for an Unresponsive Victim

R = Responsive? Tap shoulder and shout, "Are you OK?" Check for breathing and gasping.
If unresponsive and gasping or not breathing: Go to next step (A). Gasping is a sign of cardiac arrest.

If unresponsive and breathing normally: Place victim in recovery position (on victim's side with lower arm in front of body) **Figure 2-1** . For a suspected spinal injury, extend arm above head and roll body to the side so victim's head rests on extended arm.

If breath sounds are abnormal **Table 2-3** , monitor the breathing.

A = Activate EMS. Call 9-1-1.
If you are alone: Immediately call 9-1-1 (EMS) and get AED, if available. Then, return to the victim to attach and use AED.

If second rescuer is available: While one calls 9-1-1 and gets an AED, if available, the other goes to steps (P) and (C).

P = Position victim on back, on a flat, firm surface.

C = Chest compressions. Push hard and fast.
Place the heel of your hand in center of chest with the other hand on top and fingers interlaced. Push down on chest at least 2" (adults) and about 2" (children aged 1 to puberty). Allow chest to recoil completely before next compression. Deliver compressions at a rate of at least 100 per minute.

A = Airway open.
Open the victim's airway using the head tilt-chin lift method **Figure 2-2** .

B = Breaths.
Pinch the victim's nose and make an airtight seal. Give two breaths (1 second each) that make the chest rise.

D = Defibrillation.
Use the AED as soon as possible. Expose the chest, turn on the AED, and attach appropriate pads. Follow voice directions.

Table 2-3 Abnormal Breathing Sounds

Breath Sound	Potential Cause
Snoring	Tongue—If victim is unresponsive, his or her tongue may obstruct the airway, causing snoring noises.
Gurgling	Fluids in throat—Consider blood or vomit in the throat.
Stridor	Partial blockage—Consider an allergic reaction or foreign body obstruction.
Wheezing	Spasm or partial obstruction in the lungs—Consider allergic reaction or asthma attack.
Gasping respirations	Irregular breathing pattern common after the heart has stopped.

skill drill

2-1   Head-to-Toe Survey

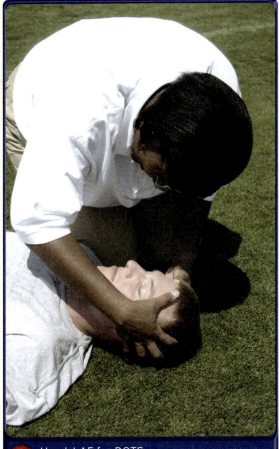

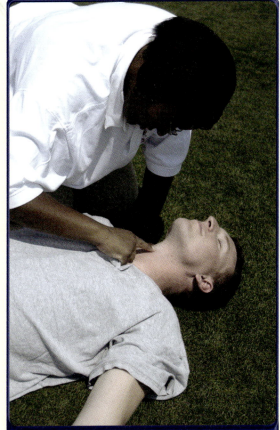

1 *Head:* LAF for DOTS.
Compare the pupils; they should be the same size. Unequal pupils suggest head injury.
Check the ears and nose for clear or blood-tinged fluid. Fluid or blood from the ears or nose suggest a head injury.
Check the mouth for objects that could block the airway, such as broken teeth or a loosened mouth guard.
Check skin color and temperature **Table 2-4** . Deformity of the face or head suggest a serious injury. Do not remove an athlete's helmet if a serious injury is suspected.

2 *Neck:* LAF for DOTS. Swelling or deformity in the neck suggest a potentially serious problem and may obstruct the airway. If a neck injury is suspected, provide manual spinal stabilization until help arrives. You may instruct a bystander to perform this procedure while you complete the assessment.

skill drill

2-1   Head-to-Toe Survey (continued)

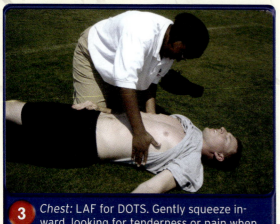

3 *Chest:* LAF for DOTS. Gently squeeze inward, looking for tenderness or pain when the victim inhales. Pain on inhalation suggests rib cage injury.

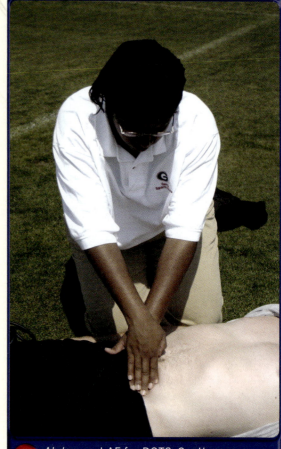

4 *Abdomen:* LAF for DOTS. Gently compress the four quadrants **Figure 2-3** of the abdomen looking for pain when you press or release. Pain when pressing down or releasing suggests internal injury.

skill drill

2-1   Head-to-Toe Survey (continued)

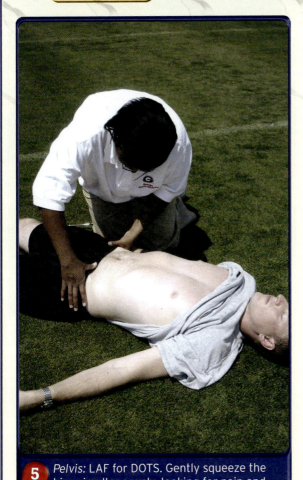

5 *Pelvis:* LAF for DOTS. Gently squeeze the hips simultaneously, looking for pain and deformity. Pain when squeezing the pelvis suggests pelvis fracture.
Back: LAF for DOTS. If necessary, and you do not suspect a spinal injury, roll the victim onto his or her side to assess the back for open wounds. **Do not roll a victim with a suspected spinal injury.**

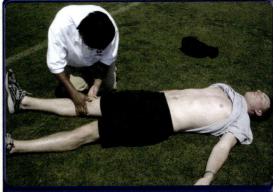

6 *Extremities:* Check both arms and legs for DOTS, circulation, sensation, movement, and range of motion (if the athlete is conscious and has only a localized injury). Check for a medical ID bracelet. Compare one side with the other. Try to determine if the athlete is not moving secondary to pain or true paralysis. Lack of sensation or weakness suggests a spinal injury.

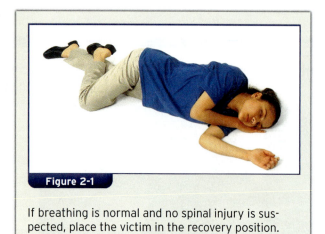

Figure 2-1

If breathing is normal and no spinal injury is suspected, place the victim in the recovery position.

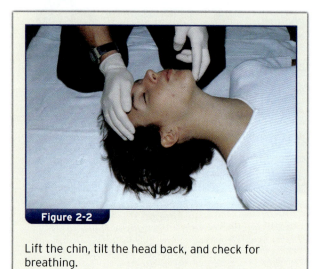

Figure 2-2

Lift the chin, tilt the head back, and check for breathing.

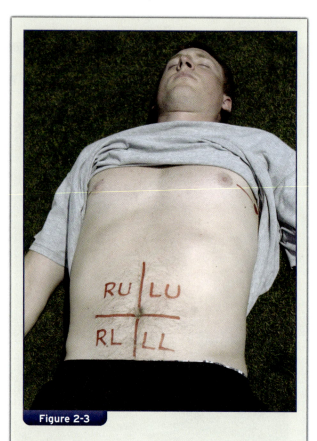

Figure 2-3

All four quadrants of the abdomen—upper right, lower right, lower left, and upper left—should be checked during the head-to-toe survey.

Table 2-4 Skin Temperature and Moisture

Skin Condition	Potential Cause
Warm and dry	Normal
Warm and moist	Exposed to hot environment, heat exhaustion, high fever
Hot and dry	Heat stroke, high fever
Cool and moist	Poor circulation, blood loss, heart problem
Cool and dry	Exposed to cold and losing heat

Not all victims require a complete head-to-toe survey, but only an assessment of the injured area. If the coach is comfortable that the injury is localized (eg, the athlete was running and twisted his or her ankle), assess the area of injury only. If the mechanism of injury is unclear or the coach has reason to believe that multiple injuries are present, perform a complete head-to-toe survey prior to moving the victim.

Circulation

Check the blood flow (*circulation*) in an arm by feeling for a pulse at the wrist; for a leg, feel for a pulse between the inside ankle knob (*malleous*) and Achilles tendon. An absent pulse demands immediate medical care.

Sensation and Movement

Check a victim's sensation by asking if he or she feels the squeezing of his or her fingers and toes. If the victim cannot feel the squeezing, consider that nerve damage has occurred. Movement can be evaluated in the upper extremity by asking the victim to squeeze the coach's hands, and in the lower extremity by asking the victim to press their foot down against a hand. Disturbance in sensation or movement may indicate serious injury.

Range-of-Motion Testing

If the injury is localized to a specific joint and the coach is comfortable that no other area is injured,
the use of the DOTS exam could be followed by range-of-motion (ROM) testing. *ROM testing* involves gently moving a joint through its normal motion and looking for a painful response or limited motion. If pain or limited motion is encountered, stop the test and seek medical care. Do not perform ROM testing if a fracture, dislocation, or other serious injury to the joint is suspected, or if the area has significant swelling. Do not perform ROM testing in an unresponsive victim.

SAMPLE History

Talk to a responsive victim and try to determine what may be injured. Perform the SAMPLE history before and during the head-to-toe survey in responsive victims **Table 2-5**. In confused or unresponsive victims, try to obtain a SAMPLE history from medical forms, bystanders, and other athletes.

Modifying the Assessment for Athletes

Perform an initial check for all sick or injured athletes. In an awake and speaking victim, the initial check is assumed to be within normal limits. Additional intervention and evaluation depends on whether the victim is injured or ill and responsive or unresponsive. **Table 2-6** describes several sequences to follow to evaluate different victims.

Table 2-5 SAMPLE History	
S = Symptoms	Where do you hurt? What is the problem? (Known as the chief complaint)
A = Allergies	Allergies to insects, medications, or food?
M = Medications currently taking	Prescription, OTCs, herbs, or vitamins?
P = Pertinent past medical problems	Recent medical problems? (Has this happened before?)
L = Last oral intake	What, when, how much? Coaches also should consider the use of illicit drugs, performance-enhancing substances, and sexual enhancement drugs and/or alcohol.
E = Events leading to injury or illness	Is this an illness or an injury? What was the mechanism of injury? Did you see the injury? Can other players, coaches, or bystanders describe the injury? Were symptoms present prior to the current problem?

Table 2-6 Sequence of Victim Assessment

Injured Victim			Ill Victim	
Unresponsive	Responsive		Unresponsive	Responsive
	Injured with significant cause of injury	Injured without significant cause of injury and a localized problem		
•Initial check •Head-to-toe survey using LAF for DOTS •SAMPLE history from others	•Initial check •Head-to-toe survey using LAF for DOTS •SAMPLE history from victim	•Initial check •Examine chief complaint •SAMPLE history from victim	•Initial check •Head-to-toe survey using LAF for DOTS •SAMPLE history from others	•Initial check •SAMPLE history from victim •Examine chief complaint

It is important to assess and reassess the level of responsiveness in injured athletes. Always explain the procedures being done and what is about to be done.

▶ Getting Help

When an athlete is injured, the coach must decide if immediate medical care (calling 9-1-1 or the local emergency number) or follow-up medical care (doctor evaluation) is required. Although common sense should be the guide, keep in mind that it is always best to make conservative decisions and act in the best interest of the athlete.

The following serious signs and symptoms indicate the need for immediate medical care. Immediate medical care can be obtained by calling 9-1-1 or the local emergency number.

- Unresponsive victim (or victim becomes unresponsive in the coach's care)
- Difficulty breathing, shortness of breath
- Chest or abdominal pain or pressure
- Fainting, sudden dizziness, weakness
- Changes in vision
- Confusion or changes in mental status

- Any sudden or severe pain
- Uncontrolled bleeding
- Severe or persistent vomiting or diarrhea
- Coughing or vomiting blood
- Suicidal or homicidal feelings
- Suspected spinal injuries
- If a victim cannot move without aggravating an injury

Call or direct someone to call 9-1-1 or the local emergency number immediately when an athlete has any of the problems identified in the list. The person who responds to the call will be an emergency medical services (EMS) dispatcher. The dispatcher will ask the person making the call:

- Their name
- The phone number from which they are calling
- The exact location of the emergency
- The nature of the emergency
- The number of athletes who are injured or ill

Speak clearly; once the dispatcher knows what has happened, he or she usually will be able to tell what needs to be done for the athlete until the ambulance arrives. Be sure to have someone meet the ambulance at its anticipated arrival location (the lo-

TIP

Do not hang up the telephone until the EMS dispatcher hangs up.

cation given to the 9-1-1 dispatcher) so that person can direct EMS personnel to the exact location of the injured athlete. Many times, large fields, gymnasiums, and other sporting complexes have many entrances and are so large that EMS crews waste valuable time looking for the victim.

Other instances of illness or injury require medical intervention but the need may not be immediate. In some situations (for example, a dislocated finger), a coach may recommend the victim be driven to the hospital by his or her parents. In some situations, a coach may recommend the victim see his or her own doctor prior to further participation in team events (in youth athletics, this recommendation must be made to the parents). If there is resistance to seeking care, the coach should require a written return-to-play note from a doctor prior to allowing the athlete to resume practicing or playing with the team. If the coach is unsure of the type of care required and a doctor is unavailable, never hesitate to go to the nearest emergency room.

Situations in which the coach may need an athlete to seek additional medical care:

- If they think a wound requires stitches
- If an athlete has a swollen/tender joint or is unable to move a joint
- If an athlete cannot bear weight on a joint
- If an athlete has a symptom of a head injury/concussion
- If an athlete appears unusually tired or weak
- If an athlete requires more than basic first aid for an injury
- If an athlete does not respond to prescribed or over-the-counter (OTC) medications
- If the coach is not comfortable placing the athlete in a competitive situation
- If an athlete has significant unexplained weight loss or weight gain

▶ The Decision to Return to Play

Return to play is the process of deciding when an injured or ill athlete can safely return to practice or competition. Although return-to-play decisions should be made by the athlete's doctor, the coach commonly is forced to make this decision on his or her own, in a short period time, and without medical consultation.

Many times an injured athlete is merely shaken up after a rough play or hard hit. No matter how minor an injury initially appears, if it caused stoppage of play, the coach should evaluate the athlete before allowing him or her to return to the competition. Many league rules require an injured player to sit out for a specified period of time if their apparent injury caused stoppage of play. A coach should be familiar with rules particular to his or her organization.

If there is any question regarding the severity of the injury, the athlete should not be moved until the coach performs an initial survey and a head-to-toe survey. If injury is noted, the victim should be treated according to first-aid protocols. If the injury appears minor or nonexistent, the victim can be assisted to the sidelines for further evaluation and treatment or a period of rest. Once the victim is off the field, the head-to-toe survey may be indicated (or repeated if already performed on the field). If the injury can be localized, a regional examination should suffice. If no injury is observed, the athlete often can return to play after a few minutes of rest.

At more competitive levels, coaches may be hesitant to make a decision that restricts a player from participating. Acting in the best welfare of the athlete and using their best judgment is the safest method to protect the athlete from further injury as well as protecting the coach from liability. Although this may conflict with immediate team goals, most would agree that the health of the athlete is of primary concern. If a coach has any doubt regarding the extent of the athlete's injuries, he or she should keep the athlete out of the competition and insist on a medical evaluation. A coach should never allow external pressures to dictate decisions that are not in the best interest of the athlete's health and well-being. A coach will never be wrong for making a conservative decision to keep the athlete off the field, but he or she will be faulted if they allow an injured player to return to play if that decision results in further aggravation to the injury.

Sometimes a busy coach may leave the return-to-play decision to the athlete or base the decision on the athlete's description of his or her current symptoms (or lack of them). Some simple procedures could be used to determine if an athlete is fit and ready to return to play. It should be reiterated that return to play is a medical decision, and although these tests may help a coach rule out significant problems and restrictions, only trained medical providers should be relied on to make the final decision. Tests to evaluate mental status, range of motion, strength, and respiratory status of an athlete provide useful information regarding his or her ability to participate. Coaches should strictly adhere to concussion/head injury guidelines. Creative exercises or activities that emulate the activities the athlete will be performing in the competition and place stress on the injured area should be performed prior to the athlete returning to competition. Activities such as squats, push-ups, hopping on one foot, and short sprints are easy to perform and can be tailored to the athlete, the sport, and the position the athlete plays.

If the softball player at the beginning of the chapter is able to hop on the injured ankle and run some sprints without pain or disability, she is likely ready to return to play.

Any injury that requires care beyond basic first-aid procedures dictates medical clearance prior to returning to play. Common situations that require medical clearance include an athlete who:

- Has a sign or symptom of a head injury or concussion
- Suffered from a heat-related illness (beyond basic heat cramps)
- Suffered symptoms of dehydration
- Recently suffered from infectious mononucleosis
- Required medical care after an injury or illness
- A coach, parent, or the athlete feels he or she is unfit to return to normal playing or practice routines

Medical clearance should be specific to the sport and athlete (eg, "Chris can return to playing soccer as of this date without limitation."). Sometimes, doctors will allow a player to return on a progressive schedule ("Chris can return to practice but body contact should be restricted. He will be reevaluated in our office on Tuesday.").

Although every situation is unique, common sense sometimes dictates return-to-play decisions. League administrators should make every attempt to limit the coach's liability for making return-to-play decisions by establishing strict evidence-based return-to-play guidelines and enforcing adherence by their coaching staff.

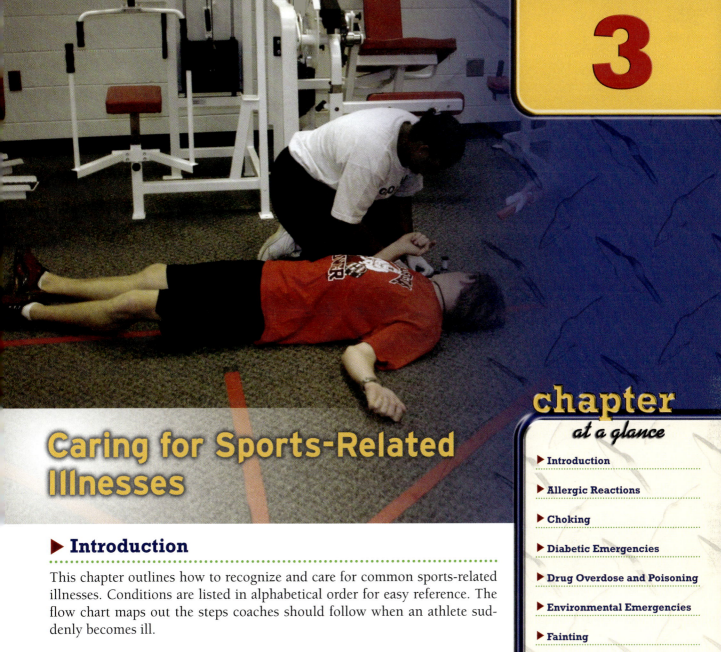

Caring for Sports-Related Illnesses

▶ Introduction

This chapter outlines how to recognize and care for common sports-related illnesses. Conditions are listed in alphabetical order for easy reference. The flow chart maps out the steps coaches should follow when an athlete suddenly becomes ill.

▶ Allergic Reactions

In victims with itchy skin, hives, rash, shortness of breath, swollen tongue, or tightness in the throat or chest, consider an allergic reaction. It should be noted that although many allergic reactions are minor, some allergic reactions progress rapidly and can quickly become life threatening.

To care for an athlete with an allergic reaction:

1. Remove the athlete from competition.
2. If the athlete's breathing is affected:
   a. Ask the athlete if he or she has a doctor-prescribed epinephrine auto-injector. If so, assist him or her in using it.
   b. Call 9-1-1 or the local emergency phone number. The athlete may be in a life-threatening situation.

chapter
at a glance

▶ **Introduction**

▶ **Allergic Reactions**

▶ **Choking**

▶ **Diabetic Emergencies**

▶ **Drug Overdose and Poisoning**

▶ **Environmental Emergencies**

▶ **Fainting**

▶ **Heart (Cardiac) Problems**

▶ **Hyperventilation Syndrome**

▶ **Motionless Athlete**

▶ **Seizures**

▶ **Shortness of Breath (Asthma and Other Breathing Problems)**

▶ **Unresponsiveness**

▶ **Vomiting**

Sudden Illness

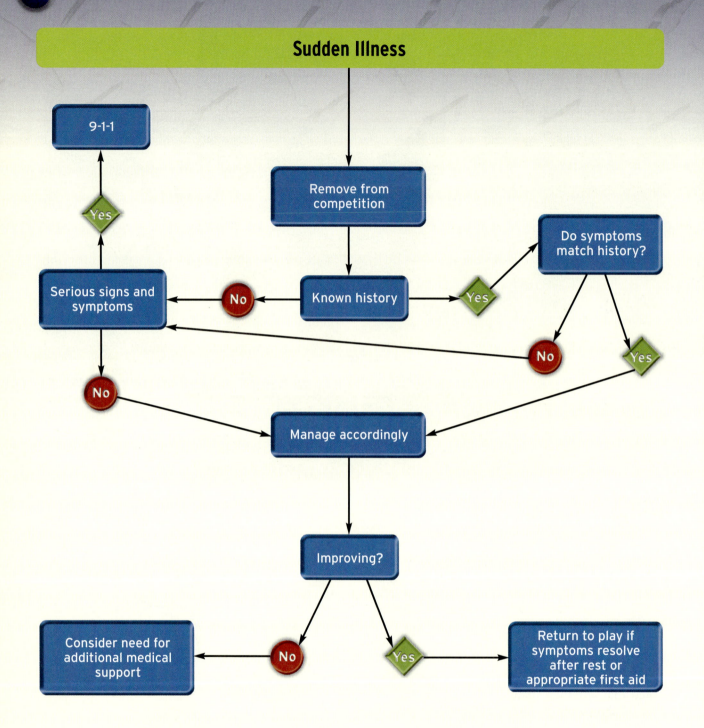

3. Try to determine the cause and seek medical care if the condition worsens.
4. For minor reactions, a doctor may recommend an antihistamine medication or hydrocortisone cream application

▶ Choking

Suspect choking in victims who suddenly cannot speak or cough or who present with the universal choking sign **Figure 3-1**. Consider food (if applicable), the athlete's mouth guard, or blood or fluid collected in the throat as possible obstructions.

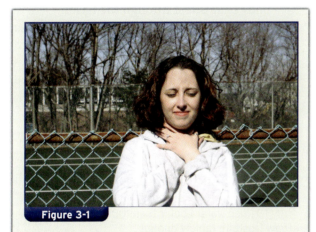

Figure 3-1

A choking athlete may use the universal distress signal for choking.

To care for an alert athlete who is choking:
1. Ask the athlete, "Are you choking?" A choking athlete cannot breathe, talk, cry, or cough.
2. Coaches should position themselves behind the athlete and place their hands above and next to the navel to give abdominal thrusts (also called the *Heimlich maneuver*).
3. Give quick inward and upward abdominal thrusts.
4. Continue abdominal thrusts until the object is expelled or the athlete becomes unresponsive. If the victim is unresponsive, give CPR with the additional step of looking into the mouth for an object before giving the two breaths and if seen, removing it.
5. Direct someone to call 9-1-1 or the local emergency number.

See Chapter 7 for more information on caring for someone who is choking.

▶ Diabetic Emergencies

If an athlete with a known history of diabetes has altered mental status, unusual behavior, or suddenly becomes unresponsive, the athlete may be experiencing a diabetic emergency. To care for an athlete with a known diabetic condition:
1. Check the level of responsiveness. The athlete may appear disoriented, may be staggering, or may be unresponsive.
2. If awake and responsive, check for the ability to swallow. Ask him or her to swallow and cough.
3. If the athlete is alert and can swallow, give food or drink containing sugar (eg, table sugar, nondiet soda, or fruit juice). It is always safe to administer sugar to a diabetic patient in an emergency situation. If the symptoms are caused by high blood glucose, the slight rise resulting from giving more sugar will not cause harm. Conversely, withholding sugar from a diabetic victim suffering from low blood glucose could have grave consequences.
4. If the athlete is not better in 15 minutes, give additional sugar and seek immediate medical care if there is no improvement.
5. Do not give an unresponsive victim (or a victim unable to consciously swallow) anything by mouth.
6. If the victim is unresponsive, support the airway using the head tilt–chin lift maneuver, and await EMS arrival.
7. Perform CPR protocols as indicated.

▶ Drug Overdose and Poisoning

If an athlete is unresponsive without a known or suspected cause, suspect a drug overdose or poisoning. Victims of drug overdose and poisoning may have abnormal behavior, drowsiness, hyperactivity, flushed face, unexplained high body temperature, rash, or itching. Also consider a drug overdose in victims with unexplained nausea and vomiting, abnormal breath odors, or other unexplained symptoms, or if others suggest the possibility of illicit drug or alcohol use. Always consider the misuse of prescription drugs, performance-enhancing substances, and alcohol.

To care for a victim with a suspected drug overdose or poisoning:

1. Evaluate and reevaluate responsiveness.
2. Determine the age and weight of the victim.
3. Determine what was ingested, how much was ingested, and when it was ingested.
4. If unresponsive, perform CPR protocols as needed.
5. Contact Poison Control (1-800-222-1222) and seek immediate medical care.
6. Do not give the victim anything by mouth.

▶ Environmental Emergencies

Cold-Related Emergencies

Consider hypothermia when an athlete's behavior and the weather conditions (cold and/or rain) suggest the possibility of abnormal loss of heat. The athlete may be acting strangely and shivering. A hypothermia victim may have been immersed in water or had a prolonged exposure to rain or dampness, may have been improperly dressed, sweating excessively, competing in a wet uniform or have low body fat or muscle mass (consider in young, thin athletes). It is important to keep in mind that hypothermia can occur any time of the year.

Suspect frostbite in below-freezing climates or if athletes are exposed to subfreezing temperatures for prolonged periods. Frostbite commonly affects the hands, ears, nose, and feet. Complaints of cold, numbness, or stinging in any of these areas often indicate frostbite. The frostbitten part may appear waxy, white, and swollen and may be tender to touch. To care for an athlete who is affected by hypothermia or frostbite:

1. Stop the heat loss. Handle the athlete gently and remove him or her from the cold environment.
2. Replace any wet clothing with dry clothing or blankets.
3. Cover the athlete's head. Fifty percent of body heat is lost through the head.
4. Do not try to rewarm a suspected frostbitten area. Treatment is best done in a medical facility.
5. If hypothermia or frostbite is suspected, seek immediate medical care.

In The News

A young female softball player was treated by paramedics for hypothermia during an evening autumn game. The paramedics immediately suspected hypothermia as they arrived on the scene to see fans wrapped in sweaters, blankets, and wool caps while the girls were playing in summer uniforms. The temperature was 48 degrees Fahrenheit and the air was moist.

CAUTION

In Cases of Frostbite

DO NOT use water hotter than 108° F—burns can result.

DO NOT use water cooler than 100° F—it will not thaw frostbite rapidly enough.

DO NOT break any blisters.

DO NOT rub or massage the affected part—ice crystals can be pushed into body cells, rupturing them.

DO NOT rub the affected part with ice or snow.

DO NOT rewarm the part with a heating pad, hot-water bottle, stove, sunlamp, radiator, or exhaust pipe or over a fire. Excessive temperatures cannot be controlled, and burns can result.

DO NOT allow the victim to drink alcoholic beverages. Alcohol dilates blood vessels and causes loss of body heat.

DO NOT allow the victim to smoke. Smoking constricts blood vessels, thus impairing circulation.

DO NOT rewarm if there is any possibility of refreezing.

DO NOT allow the thawed part to refreeze because the ice crystals formed will be larger and more damaging. If refreezing is likely or even possible, it is better to leave the affected part frozen.

Heat-Related Emergencies

Consider heat cramps or heat exhaustion in hot and humid weather conditions and when an athlete appears to be abnormally weak, sweating excessively, and/or complains of abnormal muscle cramping or is experiencing nausea.

> **TIP**
>
> **Dehydration in Athletes**
>
> Proper hydration is critical for those participating in sports and exercise. Water is an essential nutrient for important life-sustaining functions of the body and is required for optimal performance. The loss of fluids through sweating (even in cooler climates), vomiting, or diarrhea could cause dehydration and result in symptoms similar to heat exhaustion or heat stroke.
>
> Coaches should be aware of temperature and humidity levels and plan accordingly. They should ensure athletes are properly hydrated before, during, and after events. Coaches should educate their athletes about hydration and reinforce proper hydration methods throughout the season.

To care for an athlete affected by the heat:

1. Heat cramps: Muscle cramping that commonly affects the legs
   a. Have the athlete stop the activity.
   b. Move the athlete to a cool place.
   c. Give water and/or a commercial electrolyte drink.
   d. Gently stretch the cramping muscles.
   e. Do not massage the cramping muscles.
2. Heat exhaustion: Sweating, headache, nausea, dizziness or fainting (resulting from activity in a hot and/or humid environment)
   a. Move the athlete to a cool place.
   b. Have the athlete lie down and raise the legs 6 to 12 inches.
   c. Remove any excess or restrictive clothing/equipment.
   d. If the athlete is alert and not nauseated, have him or her drink water and/or a commercial electrolyte drink.
   e. Sponge with cool water or fan the athlete.

   f. Call 9-1-1 or the local emergency number if the athlete does not improve within 30 minutes.
   g. The athlete should not return to play for 24 hours and should be advised to increase their water and electrolytes for the next 24 hours.
3. Heat stroke: Extremely hot skin, altered mental status (confusion, agitation to unresponsiveness). This condition is rare in young athletes.
   a. Call 9-1-1 or the local emergency number.
   b. Move the athlete to a cool place.
   c. Remove any excess clothing.
   d. Keep the head and shoulders slightly raised.
   e. Quickly cool the victim by any means possible. Place ice packs in the armpits, sides of neck, and groin. Spraying with water and fanning works in low-humidity conditions.

▶ Fainting

To care for an athlete who feels faint or has fainted:

1. Have the athlete lie down and raise the legs 6 to 12 inches.
2. Monitor responsiveness and breathing.
3. Loosen any restrictive clothing.
4. Apply a cool, wet cloth to the athlete's forehead and neck.
5. If the athlete is uninjured, assist him or her in slowly sitting up.
6. Be sure to report the episode to the athlete's parents.
7. Consider the causes of the fainting. If nothing is obvious, seek medical care.

> **CAUTION**
>
> **If an Athlete Feels Faint or Has Fainted**
> - **DO NOT** splash or pour water onto an athlete's face to revive him or her.
> - **DO NOT** use smelling salts or ammonia inhalants.
> - **DO NOT** slap the athlete's face.
> - **DO NOT** give the athlete anything to drink until he or she can sit fully upright and swallow.

▶ Heart (Cardiac) Problems

Although rare, cardiac problems can occur in young athletes. The presence of a sideline automated external defibrillator (AED) should be encouraged at all levels of athletic competition. Cardiac problems should be considered in any athlete with a known history of a heart condition or any athlete with unexplained chest tightness or pain or who suddenly collapses. It also is not uncommon for coaches, referees, and bystanders to suffer from cardiac events during a sporting event.

The possible signs and symptoms of a heart attack include:

- Pressure, squeezing, heaviness, or pain in the center of the chest that lasts more than a few minutes (pain may come and go).
- Pain reported to be similar to a previous heart attack.
- Pain may spread to the arms (especially the left), jaw, or neck.
- If any of the following occur in addition to the previous complaints:
  - Nausea
  - Sweating
  - Dizziness
  - Shortness of breath

TIP

Suspect a heart problem in any victim who suddenly collapses without other reasonable causes.

To care for an athlete with a suspected cardiac problem:

1. Have the athlete stop all activity immediately.
2. Place him or her in a comfortable seated or half-sitting position.
3. Loosen restrictive clothing.
4. Call 9-1-1 or the local emergency number.
5. Allow the athlete to take one aspirin (if not allergic).
6. Allow the athlete to take medications (such as nitroglycerin) if instructed to do so by

their doctor. Do not use anyone else's medication and do not give unresponsive victims anything by mouth.

7. If the athlete is unresponsive, use CPR/AED protocols.

▶ Hyperventilation Syndrome

Hyperventilation syndrome is a condition of rapid breathing and is not related to an underlying medical condition. A coach should suspect hyperventilation syndrome in victims who are anxious and breathing rapidly following a stressful event or those with a history of anxiety and/or hyperventilation syndrome. Always rule out more serious breathing problems (such as asthma) in a victim with abnormal breathing.

1. Determine the cause of hyperventilation.
   a. Did something happen to upset the victim?
   b. Has the athlete had a similar episode in the past?
2. Rule out other breathing emergencies (such as an asthma attack).
3. Talk to the athlete in a reassuring and calm voice.
4. Encourage the athlete to take long, slow breaths and to hold each breath before slowly exhaling.
5. Call 9-1-1 or the local emergency number if the athlete has a severe or prolonged episode.

▶ Motionless Athlete

Follow these steps to care for an athlete who is not moving:

1. See if the athlete is responsive by tapping him or her on the shoulder and loudly asking, "Are you OK?"
2. If the athlete does not respond, call or direct someone to call 9-1-1 or the local emergency number.
3. Tilt the athlete's head back and lift the chin (even for those with a suspected spinal injury unless trained in the jaw-thrust maneuver).
4. Check for breathing by looking at the rise and fall of the chest, listening for breath

sounds, and feeling for breaths with the cheek (take 5 to 10 seconds).

5. If the athlete is not breathing, give two breaths (each lasting 1 second) **Figure 3-2**.

6. Give 30 chest compressions followed by two breaths.

Suspect absence of breathing in an athlete who is unresponsive, lacks an effective rise and fall of the chest, or appears abnormally blue or pale in color and lacks signs of life.

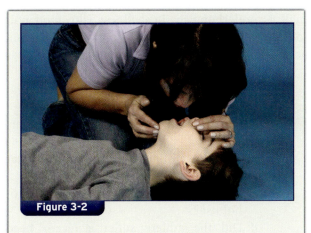

Figure 3-2

If the athlete is not breathing, give two slow breaths.

▶ Seizures

Suspect a seizure in athletes with a history of seizures or epilepsy and in athletes with a recent head injury. The seizure victim will be shaking and twitching uncontrollably. Be aware of absence seizures, which are most common in children. To care for an athlete experiencing a seizure:

1. Remove nearby objects to prevent injury.
2. Remove constricting or tight clothing.
3. Do not try to restrain the athlete having a seizure. Do not place any object between the teeth.
4. Roll the athlete onto his or her side immediately after the seizure to help keep the airway clear.
5. Call 9-1-1 or the local emergency number.

TIP

Absence Seizures
This type of seizure is more common in children and also is known as a petit mal seizure. It is characterized by a blank stare lasting for a short time. It may be accompanied by rapid blinking and/or chewing movements. The child is unaware of what is going on and usually returns to full awareness quickly.

CAUTION

New onset of seizures always requires immediate medical care.

▶ Shortness of Breath (Asthma and Other Breathing Problems)

Consider asthma or an allergic reaction if the victim reports unexplained shortness of breath, fails to recover from exercise, appears unexpectedly anxious or struggling to catch breath, uses a hand-held inhaler repeatedly, continuously removes the mouth guard and/or facemask between plays, or becomes unresponsive. Breathing problems should always be considered serious until proven otherwise. To care for an athlete with asthma or a breathing problem:

1. Have the athlete sit upright or in the most comfortable position.
2. If the athlete has a doctor-prescribed, hand-held inhaler, have him or her:
   a. Exhale deeply.
   b. Place his or her lips around the inhaler's opening.
   c. Depress the inhaler while inhaling deeply.
   d. Hold his or her breath for several seconds.
   e. Encourage the athlete to perform this slowly to ensure the medication is

entering all the lung fields. The athlete should then exhale through pursed lips.

    f. This may be repeated a second time.

3. Call 9-1-1 or the local emergency number if the condition does not improve.

TIP

It is quite common for an athlete to "get their wind knocked out" and appear to have shortness of breath for several seconds. Any blow to the abdomen can cause a spasm in the large muscle located between the abdominal cavity and the chest cavity called the *diaphragm*. When the diaphragm is in spasm, it is difficult for the athlete to catch his or her breath. This problem will resolve usually on its own with a few minutes of rest. Some recommend having the athlete lie down and lift his or her arms over their chest to expand the chest cavity (hold-up position). This is okay as long as no injury is present. If shortness of breath does not resolve after a few minutes or other injuries are present, call 9-1-1 or the local emergency number.

▶ Unresponsiveness

Consider all potential medical and traumatic causes of unresponsiveness. To care for an unresponsive athlete:

1. Open the airway (use head tilt–chin lift, unless trauma is suspected and the coach is trained in the jaw-thrust maneuver) and check for breathing.
2. If the athlete is not breathing, place them on their back and begin CPR protocols.
3. If the athlete is breathing, place them on their side in the recovery position (if no trauma is suspected; if trauma is suspected, leave them on their back and provide manual spinal stabilization).
4. Continuously reassess the level of responsiveness.

CAUTION

DO NOT leave an unresponsive athlete on his or her back if vomiting.

---

5. Perform a head-to-toe survey and treat any apparent problems.
6. Call 9-1-1 or the local emergency number.

▶ Vomiting

If an athlete is vomiting, consider potential causes such as underlying medical illness (flu, food poisoning, and stomach virus), anxiety, drug ingestion, or internal injuries. To care for a vomiting athlete:

1. Remove the athlete from competition.
2. Have the victim sit down and rest.
3. Try to determine the cause of the vomiting.
    a. Did the athlete overexert him- or herself?
    b. Did the athlete eat something earlier that may have caused any problems?
    c. Is there any possibility of drug or alcohol use?
    d. Did the athlete suffer a recent head injury?
    e. Was there any trauma that could have caused internal injuries?
    f. Does the athlete appear sick (feverish, pale, clammy)?
4. Seek medical care if:
    a. Blood or dark fluid is seen in the vomit.
    b. The victim complains of persistent abdominal pain.
    c. The victim feels faint when standing.
    d. Projectile vomiting occurs.
    e. The vomiting follows a recent head injury.
5. Do not let the athlete return to competition until nausea and vomiting have stopped or until the athlete is cleared by a doctor.
6. Give the victim small amounts of water to sip.

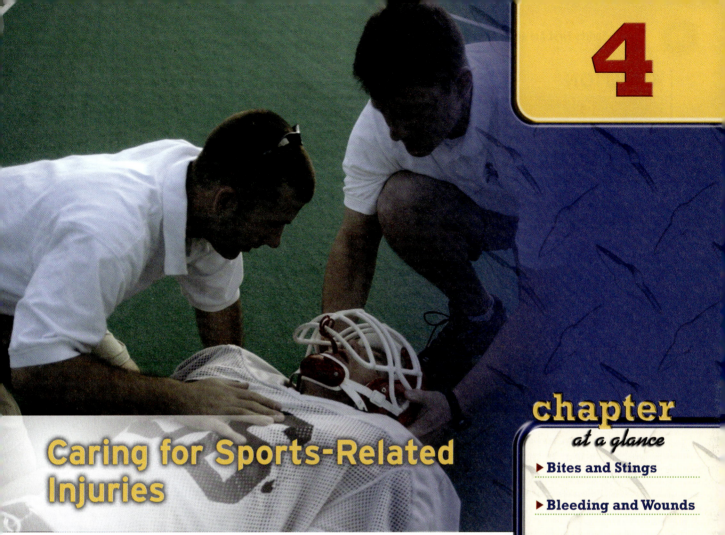

Caring for Sports-Related Injuries

▶ Bites and Stings

Suspect an insect sting if the victim experiences sudden sharp, localized pain, redness, or swelling without other explanation. To care for an alert athlete with a sting:

1. See if a stinger is embedded in the athlete's skin. Only honeybees leave an embedded stinger, and it may have a venom sac attached.
2. If a stinger is found, scrape it out with a fingernail or the edge of a credit card.
3. Wash the affected area with soap and water.
4. Apply an ice pack or cold compress for 15 to 20 minutes.
5. Observe the athlete for 30 minutes for signs of an allergic reaction.
6. An antihistamine medication may be recommended by a doctor.
7. If the athlete's breathing is affected:
   a. Ask the athlete if he or she has a doctor-prescribed epinephrine auto-injector. If so, assist him or her in using it.
   b. Call 9-1-1 or the local emergency phone number.

chapter
at a glance

▶ **Bites and Stings**

▶ **Bleeding and Wounds**

▶ **Blisters**

▶ **Burns**

▶ **Contusions**

▶ **Dislocations**

▶ **Drowning**

▶ **Fractures**

▶ **Sprains**

▶ **Strains**

▶ **Common Injuries by Region**

CAUTION

DO NOT pull out a honeybee stinger with a venom sac still attached to it with tweezers or your fingers; you may squeeze poisonous venom into the athlete!

▶ Bleeding and Wounds

In the course of practice or athletic competition, an athlete may sustain a wound with bleeding. To control the bleeding, press a sterile or clean article (known as a *dressing*) directly over the wound site. Many types of sterile dressings are commercially available. If no sterile dressing is available, use any clean article. A *bandage* is a clean article and is used to hold the dressing in place. Roller gauze or a folded triangular bandage (cravat) makes a great bandage to hold a dressing in place.

Most bleeding can be stopped with direct pressure and elevation. Be patient and do not remove the dressing to see if the bleeding has stopped. Table 4-1 lists types of wounds with their appearance and recommended treatment.

To care for an athlete with a major wound (significant blood flow, gaping wound):

1. Seek immediate medical care.
2. Wear medical exam gloves.
3. Cover the wound with a clean, dry cloth or a sterile dressing.
4. Press the dressing firmly against the wound for 5 to 10 minutes.
5. If bleeding continues from an arm or a leg, raise the injured area above the heart level if possible (unless a fracture or other injury is suspected), while pressing on the wound.
6. Secure a dressing snugly in place with a bandage Figure 4-1 .
7. Leave blood-soaked dressings in place. If the dressing is soaked through, apply another dressing over the blood-soaked one.

To care for an athlete with a minor wound:

1. Wear medical exam gloves.
2. Press the dressing firmly against the wound for 5 to 10 minutes.
3. Wash the wound thoroughly with soap and water.
4. Flush the inside of the wound with forceful water.

Table 4-1 Classification of Wounds

Type of Wound	Appearance	Treatment
Puncture	A sharp object that penetrates the skin deeply	Stop the bleeding. If the object is still in the wound, do not remove it; puncture wounds have a high risk of infection.
Laceration	A cut with a jagged edge	Stop the bleeding. The laceration may need stitches to prevent scarring.
Incision	A cut with a cleanly defined edge	Stop the bleeding.
Abrasion	Scraped or removed skin	Stop the bleeding. Clean the entire wound with soap and water. Consider covering the wound to prevent infection.
Avulsion/amputation	A piece of skin or body part partially or completely detaches from the body	Stop the bleeding. Secure an avulsion in place with a dressing and bandage. If an amputation occurs, find the amputated part and seek medical care.

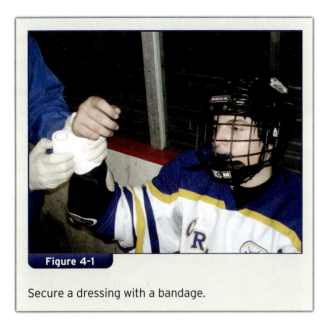

Figure 4-1

Secure a dressing with a bandage.

5. Cover the wound with a clean, dry cloth or a sterile dressing.
6. When the bleeding stops, apply an antibiotic ointment and then secure the dressing snugly in place.
7. Advise the athlete to look for signs of infection (redness, swelling, pain, tenderness) and to seek medical care if this occurs.
8. Consider the need for stitches.

Wounds that Need Suturing

Athletes commonly suffer from lacerations and open wounds that require closure by medical personnel. Determining which wounds need medical care often confuses coaches, parents, and athletes. Although each situation is unique, some general guidelines will help individuals determine when wound suturing is required, who should perform the procedure, and finally what to do if an athlete who has received stitches shows up ready to play for a practice or game.

Sutures are used in wound care to help control bleeding and help prevent unsightly scars. Situations that require suturing (or additional medical consultation) include:

- Wounds that are deeply cut that show muscle, fat, or bone

- Any wound that is gaping open and whose edges cannot be opposed
- Lacerations longer than 1 inch
- Wounds that will not stop bleeding with traditional techniques (Large wounds with uncontrolled bleeding require immediate medical care.)
- Wounds that involve joints
- Facial lacerations or lacerations in areas where a scar would be visible
- Human or animal bites
- Deep puncture wounds (or those with embedded objects)
- Wounds with jagged lacerations
- Unusually dirty wounds

Sutures should be inserted within 6 hours after the injury. If there is any delay, be sure to clean the wound thoroughly and keep it clean and moist until the athlete can see a doctor. Most wounds can be adequately sutured by emergency department doctors. Some wounds can be closed by the family doctor, though the office hours and time constraints of a private practice doctor may make the family doctor a less-than-desirable choice for this type of care. Wounds involving the face or areas where a scar would affect the athlete's appearance need expert closure by a plastic surgeon.

In recent years, there has been increased use of Steri-strips and alternative skin closure methods. Although these may be a good option, the decision to use an alternative method of skin closure should be left to a doctor. Although Steri-strips offer a comfortable alternative to stitches, they do have their limitations and potential dangers. Alternative skin closure methods should not be used by nontrained medical personnel.

When caring for a wound that has been closed with sutures:

- The wound should be kept dry for 24–48 hours.
- The athlete should be advised to apply an antibiotic cream at least two times per day or as directed by a doctor.
- The wound should be covered for at least 48 hours after the stitches are placed.
- Stitches should be removed only by trained health care professionals. Athletes should

be strongly discouraged from removing their own stitches.

- The length of time stitches should stay in place varies from 5 days to 2 weeks and should be directed by a doctor.
- Coaches should require a doctor's note stating when the athlete may return to complete activity.

Athletes should be advised to contact their doctor if any signs of infection occur. These signs include continued redness (beyond a day or two after stitches), pain or abnormal swelling in the area of the wound, red streaks around the wound, and fever.

The decision to return an athlete who has received sutures to competition is unique for each situation. Athletes should be allowed to return to play only with doctor clearance. In general, an athlete should not return to any activity for a minimum of 48 hours after stitches are placed. This time may be lengthened if the stitches are in a location where activity can aggravate the wound. The type of wound, the level of competition, the athlete's role on the team, and the age of the athlete are all factors that the athlete's doctors should be aware of when making the decision to return to play after receiving stitches. At higher levels of athletic participation, team doctors usually determine the need for stitches and the return to play. Although wound care guidelines may not be strictly followed at these levels of sports participation, their circumstances are unique and influenced by factors irrelevant to youth athletes. Most youth sport coaches should act on the conservative side when dealing with children with open wounds, and should always act in the best interest of the child. The next page features a flowchart on bleeding and wounds.

▶ Blisters

Poorly fitted equipment, old or new equipment, or improperly worn equipment are common causes of blisters. To care for an athlete with an unbroken blister:

1. Clean the area with soap and water.
2. Cut doughnut-shaped holes in several pieces of moleskin or molefoam to fit around the blister.

3. Apply a stack of several doughnut-shaped pads around the blister Figure 4-2 , place antibiotic ointment in the hole, and then cover it with an uncut gauze pad.
4. Consider removing the athlete from competition or modifying equipment.

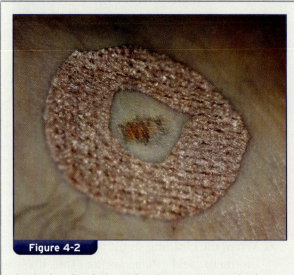

Figure 4-2

Apply doughnut-shaped pads around an unbroken blister.

To care for an athlete with a broken blister:

1. Clean the area with soap and water.
2. Apply a stack of several doughnut-shaped pads around the blister, place antibiotic ointment in the hole, and then cover it with an uncut gauze pad.
3. Advise the athlete to watch for signs of infection (redness, swelling, pain, tenderness).

▶ Burns

Burns can be classified as thermal (heat), chemical, or electrical. To care for an athlete with burns, consider the cause:

1. If due to a fire, be sure the fire is extinguished and the area is safe.
2. If due to fire or heat and the burn appears superficial (such as a sunburn):

Bleeding and Wounds

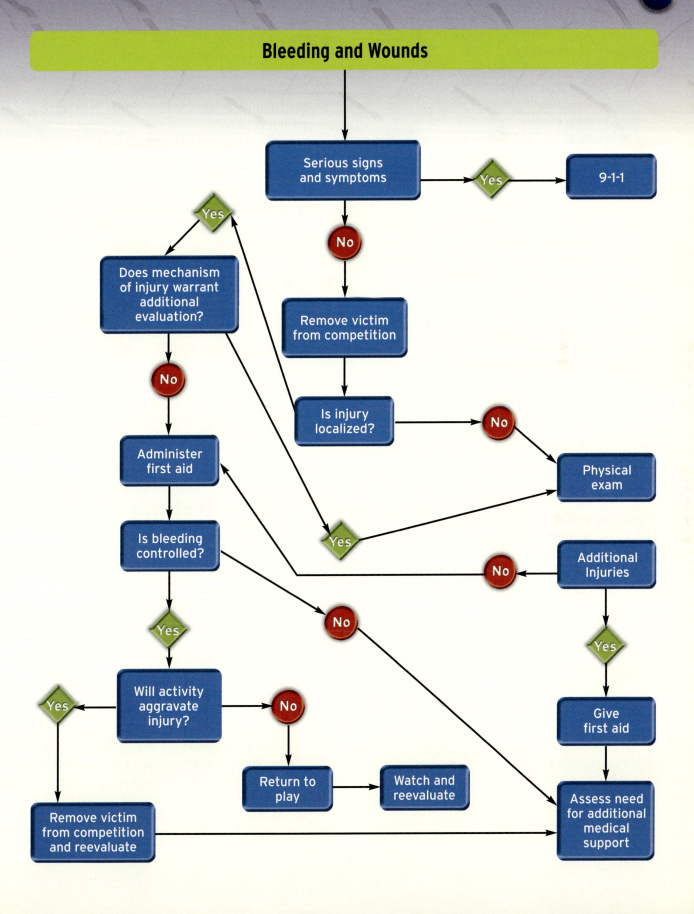

a. Apply cold compresses to the skin for 10–45 minutes.

b. Apply skin moisturizer.

c. Consider applying a nonstick dressing.

d. Consider additional medical care for pain control.

3. If due to fire and the burns appear deep or are accompanied by other injury:

a. Perform an initial check and physical assessment and manage existing injuries accordingly.

b. Remove equipment, clothing, and jewelry from the area.

c. Apply a sterile dressing or a clean cloth.

d. Seek immediate medical care.

4. If due to a chemical, beware of contact with the corrosive substance.

a. Flush the area immediately with water for 20 minutes.

b. Seek immediate medical care.

c. Remove all clothing and jewelry.

d. Do not attempt to neutralize.

5. If due to an electrical current, be sure the area is safe. Unplug, disconnect, or turn off the electrical power. If that is not possible, call 9-1-1 or the local emergency number. Never touch an energized wire, object, or victim. If the area is safe:

a. Perform an initial check and head-to-toe survey and manage existing injuries accordingly.

b. Apply CPR protocols as indicated.

c. Treat burns as if they are thermal burns.

d. Seek immediate medical care.

e. All victims of lightning injuries need medical evaluation.

TIP

Sunburn

Athletes participating in outdoor events, especially on sunny days, are always at risk of sunburn. *Sunburn* is a superficial burn and should be treated as such. Sunburn can cause considerable discomfort. It is important that athletes competing in outdoor activities are properly protected with sunscreen used appropriately for age and activity.

▶ Contusions

Suspect a *contusion* (bruise) if the victim received a direct hit producing swelling, pain and tenderness, localized tightness, or a visible bruise (can appear several hours later).

In caring for an athlete with a contusion:

1. Remove the athlete from competition.

2. Apply an ice pack for 20 minutes, three to four times daily for the next 48 hours.

3. Use an elastic bandage to apply compression to the contusion.

4. If not improving, seek medical care.

▶ Dislocations

A *dislocation* occurs when a joint becomes grossly misaligned. Dislocations can occur in any joint but are common in the shoulders, fingers and toes, knees, and ankles. Suspect a dislocation if the area is grossly deformed (compare with the other side) or if the victim has a history of dislocations. To care for an athlete with a suspected dislocation (see also Common Injuries by Region):

1. Remove the athlete from competition.

2. Apply ice to the area.

3. Splint it in the position in which it is found.

4. Discourage the athlete or others from attempting to reduce the dislocation unless directed by trained medical personnel.

▶ Drowning

Rescue the victim by throwing something that floats to them or use something to pull him or her to safety. Do not go to the victim unless trained in water rescue. Once rescued:

1. Check for unresponsiveness and breathing.

2. Be aware of potential spinal injury. If injury was not witnessed or mechanism of injury suggests potential spinal injury, use caution when establishing an airway. The head tilt–chin lift is recommended for lay rescuers not trained in the jaw-thrust maneuver.

3. Provide CPR as indicated (if trained).

4. Do not attempt methods to remove water from the victim's lungs.

5. Call 9-1-1 or the local emergency number. Near-drowning victims always need to go to the hospital.

▶ Fractures

Suspect a fracture if any of the following are recognized:

- Deformity—Compare the injured side with the uninjured side.
- Open wound—An open wound may suggest an underlying fracture. Bone ends protruding through the skin suggest a serious underlying fracture.
- Tenderness and pain—Localized tenderness over a bone or joint. The athlete will commonly protect or guard the injured area. Sometimes they will try to prevent someone from examining the area. If an athlete is apprehensive and is trying to prevent someone from examining the injury, suspect a fracture and seek medical care.
- Swelling—Compare the injured side to the noninjured side.
- An athlete reports hearing a pop, feeling a grating sensation (*crepitus*), or refuses to bear weight or use the injured area.

To care for an athlete with a suspected fracture:

1. Unless the injury is localized, be sure to complete a physical assessment prior to caring for the apparent fracture.
2. If the victim is unresponsive or a spinal or skull fracture is suspected, seek immediate medical care. Manage all other problems accordingly while minimizing movement to the victim.
3. In alert victims, immobilize the injured area with a splint:
   a. Splint it in the most comfortable position if the injury is localized and the victim is awake and alert. The victim likely will have already found the position of least pain.
   b. Splint it in the position it is found if the injury involves a joint, the victim cannot move it, or if unsure of the best position.
4. Apply ice to the injury site.

5. Cover any open wounds and stop any bleeding. If bone ends are protruding from an open fracture, do not push them back. As much as possible, splint it the way it is found and seek immediate medical care.

Applying a Splint

All fractures and dislocations should be stabilized before the victim is moved. Although athletic trainers and EMS providers have access to specialized splinting equipment, most coaches will have limited splinting supplies and lack experience in applying these devices. Minimizing the movement of the victim and the injured area until more experienced personnel arrive is often the best care a coach could provide. If no other help is imminent and it becomes necessary for the coach to apply a splint, the following information would be helpful.

The best type of splint is a rigid, inflexible device. It can be a padded board, a piece of heavy cardboard, or a commercially available SAM splint that can be molded to fit the extremity (SAM splints are inexpensive and easily fit in a team first aid kit). Whatever its construction, a rigid splint must be long enough to be secured well above and below the fracture site. A soft splint, such as a pillow or folded blanket, is useful for stabilizing many fractures, especially those involving the lower leg or the forearm. A coach can learn to use a sling and swathe to stabilize shoulder and upper extremity problems **Figure 4-3**.

An *anatomic splint* is always available because it uses the body itself as a splint. An anatomic splint is one in which the injured bone is secured to an uninjured part (for example, taping an injured finger to a noninjured finger).

Before applying a splint, cover any open wounds with a sterile dressing. If two people are present, one should support the injury site and minimize movement of the extremity until splinting is completed. When possible, place the splint materials on both sides of the injured part, especially when two bones are involved (eg, fractures involving the lower arm or lower leg). This sandwich splint prevents the injured extremity from rotating and keeps the two bones from touching. With

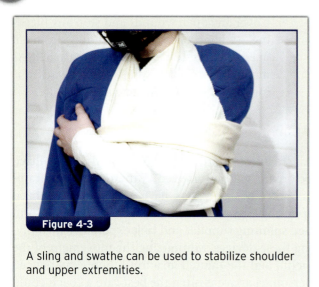

Figure 4-3

A sling and swathe can be used to stabilize shoulder and upper extremities.

rigid splints, use extra padding in natural body hollows and around any deformities. Secure the splint in place with an elastic bandage or cravat, but not so tightly that blood flow into an extremity is affected. Leave the fingers or toes exposed.

TIP

Splinting Materials

Coaches can take advantage of protective sporting gear, which often make great splinting devices.

- Pillow splint around ankle
- Blanket around forearm
- Shin pad for knee fracture
- Anatomical leg splint
- Buddy-taped finger

▶ Sprains

A *sprain* is an injury to the ligaments that surround and support a joint. Suspect a sprain if the athlete reports pain or swelling after twisting or compressing a joint or reports abnormal pain, swelling, or

pressure in a joint after a collision or fall. To care for a victim with a suspected sprain (see also Common Injuries by Region):

1. Remove the athlete from competition.
2. Apply ice for 20 minutes.
3. If a minor sprain is suspected and the injury is localized, evaluate the joint for range of motion and the ability to bear weight.
4. In minor sprains, advise the athlete to stop activity for at least 24 hours and apply RICE principles.
5. If pain, swelling, and restricted motion persist, seek medical care.
6. Sometimes it is difficult (even for trained medical personnel) to differentiate a sprain from a strain and commonly sprain/strain injuries are concurrent.

TIP

Is It Fractured or Sprained?

This is perhaps one of the most common questions medical personnel are asked by coaches, athletes, and parents. Athletes commonly injure a bone and/or joint during a practice or competition and hours later recognize increasing pain and discomfort, causing concern about the extent of the injury. There is one simple rule that everyone can apply to these types of injuries: **Unless the fractured bone segment is protruding from the skin or there is a severe deformity, the only way to detect a fracture is with an x-ray image.**

Many parents and coaches use unsubstantiated "diagnostic" methods to guess if a bone is fractured. Swelling, discoloration, and the ability or inability to move an injured area are not reliable methods of diagnosing a bone or joint injury. Such procedures often lead to sleepless nights, premature return-to-play decisions, and midnight visits to the emergency department. There is no evidence that swelling and range-of-motion features are accurate indicators of fractures. If unsettled by a joint injury, rather than delaying the treatment or worrying needlessly, get an x-ray as soon as possible.

TIP

Sprain/Strain

Although sprains always occur around a joint, a strain can occur near a joint or anywhere along a muscle. It is often difficult to differentiate a strain from a sprain and they commonly occur concurrently.

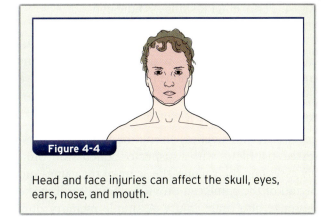

Figure 4-4

Head and face injuries can affect the skull, eyes, ears, nose, and mouth.

▶ Strains

A *strain* is an injury to the muscles or tendons that help move a joint or bone. Suspect a strain if the athlete reports sudden pain or swelling after activity. They may or may not report specific trauma prior to the injury. Occasionally, an athlete may hear a pop indicating a severe strain (or tear). To care for a victim with a suspected strain (see also Common Injuries by Region):

1. Remove the athlete from competition.
2. Apply ice to the injured area for 20 minutes.
3. In minor strains, advise the athlete to stop activity for at least 24 hours and apply RICE principles.
4. If pain, swelling, and restricted motion persist, seek medical care.
5. Sometimes it is difficult (even for trained medical personnel) to differentiate a sprain from a strain and commonly sprain/strain injuries are concurrent.

▶ Common Injuries by Region

Head and Face Injuries

Injuries to the head and face area **Figure 4-4** can affect the outer or inner aspect of the skull or both, the eyes, ears, nose, and mouth. Injuries to this area can range from minor external wounds that can be managed with basic first aid skills to serious brain trauma that requires advanced medical/surgical intervention. Helmets do not always guarantee full protection from a head injury. Head injuries can have devastating consequences and coaches must be familiar with immediate or early recognition and management.

Brain Injury

Concussion, contusion, and hematoma are common brain injuries substained by athletes. In addition to direct trauma to the head, any forceful blow to an athlete's head or body that results in rapid movement of the head can damage nerves and/or blood vessels in the brain. Bleeding within the closed skull cavity (contusion and hematoma) can produce swelling in the brain, which interferes with critical brain functions. Disruption of the nerve cells (as in a concussion) may have temporary or long-term effects on the brain.

Suspect serious brain injury (such as a contusion, hematoma, or internal bleeding) and get immediate medical care if any of the following occur after a head injury:

- Unresponsiveness
- A headache that gets worse or does not go away
- Repeated vomiting or nausea
- Convulsions or seizures
- An inability to awaken from sleep
- Dilation of one or both pupils of the eyes
- Slurred speech
- Weakness or numbness in the arms or legs
- Loss of coordination
- Increased confusion, restlessness, or agitation

To care for athlete with a suspected serious head injury:

1. **Do not move the athlete.**
2. Maintain spinal stabilization.
3. Manage other injuries accordingly.

4. Perform CPR skills as indicated.

5. Call 9-1-1 or the local emergency number.

Remember, the effects of concussions are cumulative; therefore, athletes with multiple concussions are at greater risk of serious problems if they receive another head injury.

Assessing Level of Responsiveness

Level of responsiveness should be immediately assessed in athletes with a suspected concussion. Simply assessing their name, the score of the game, and period of the game can provide clues regarding the presence of a brain injury. A simple memory quiz can be used to see if the athlete has a deficit in his or her short-term memory. Tell the athlete to remember the short statement that will be told to them and to repeat it later whenever requested. Use the statement "you can't teach an old dog new tricks." Asking the athlete to repeat this statement several times in the immediate minutes and hours following a head injury is a good way to assess the presence of a concussion. Inability to remember this statement suggests the presence of a brain injury and the need for medical follow-up.

It is important to remember that symptoms of concussion (or any head injury) could take hours or days to develop. If any of the previous signs and symptoms occurs in the hours or days following a head injury, additional medical support should be sought.

Do not allow the athlete to return to play without a doctor's clearance. It is not uncommon for an athlete with a known or suspected concussion to want to return to sports participation. In the days and weeks following a concussion, the brain is more vulnerable to "second-impact syndrome." Second-impact syndrome occurs when the brain experiences multiple impacts without complete recovery, resulting in long-term damage. It is imperative that the athlete refrain from physical activity until completely recovered. Complete recovery can be documented after appropriate neuropsychological testing and evaluation by a neurologist trained in concussion management.

Skull Fracture

A skull fracture can occur in any victim who sustains head trauma. If the athlete was wearing a helmet, be sure to inspect the helmet for damage. A damaged helmet is a strong clue for an underlying head injury. The athlete may or may not be unresponsive and may or may not have an open wound. Although skull fractures often are difficult to detect, the athlete with a skull fracture may have any of the following:

- Pain at the point of injury
- Deformity of the skull
- Bleeding or clear fluid from the ears or nose
- Discoloration around the eyes ("raccoon eyes") or behind the ears (Battle's sign) **Figure 4-5**

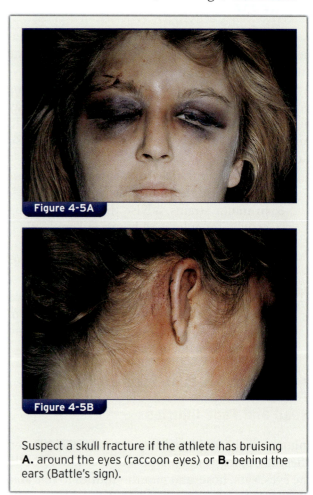

Figure 4-5A

Figure 4-5B

Suspect a skull fracture if the athlete has bruising **A.** around the eyes (raccoon eyes) or **B.** behind the ears (Battle's sign).

To care for a victim with a suspected skull fracture:

1. Consider a spinal injury. If a spinal injury is suspected, maintain manual spinal stabilization and do not move the victim.

2. If bleeding is present, apply pressure around the wound but not directly on it.
3. Apply a sterile or clean dressing.
4. Seek immediate medical care.

Scalp Wounds

Scalp wounds often appear to produce disproportionate amounts of blood. Often cleaning the area around the wound and locating the exact wound reveals a smaller, more controllable wound than expected. Once the site of bleeding is localized:

1. Control bleeding with direct pressure.
2. Once the bleeding stops, wash the wound with soap and water.
3. If a skull fracture associated with the bleeding is suspected, apply pressure on the wound's outer edges and seek immediate medical care.
4. If there is swelling and pain, apply an ice pack for 20 minutes.
5. Evaluate the need for stitches.

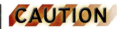

CAUTION

DO NOT apply pressure to an injured eye.

Eye Injuries

The anatomic structure of the skull and facial bones (*eye orbits*) deflects many potential eye injuries to the area surrounding the eye. In addition to caring for an injury that surrounds the eye socket, it is important to evaluate the eye itself to determine if any direct eyeball injury has occurred. To care for a direct eyeball injury:

1. If there is a loose object in the eye:
   a. Pull down the lower eyelid and have the athlete look up.
   b. If the object is seen, remove it either by flushing the eye with water or by using a clean, moist cloth or sterile dressing.
   c. Lift the upper eyelid and have the athlete look down.
   d. If the object can be seen, remove it either by flushing the eye with water or using a clean, moist cloth or sterile dressing.

   e. Seek medical care if irritation persists or it is believed the object has not been removed.
2. If there is a fixed object in the athlete's eye:
   a. Call 9-1-1 or the local emergency number.
   b. Do not remove the object.
   c. Protect the eye to prevent the object from being driven deeper.
   d. Bandaging both eyes is recommended. If one eye moves, the other eye also moves, so covering both eyes keeps the injured eye motionless. Remember, the victim now cannot see and will need assistance. Do not leave this victim alone.
   e. For a long object embedded in the eyeball, do not remove it, because blindness could result. Try to stabilize the object to prevent it from moving and causing further harm. Use bulky dressings or clean cloths to stabilize and prevent any movement of the object. Extreme care should be taken when applying the dressing to limit movement. Some recommend securing a paper cup cone over the object for protection against it being driven in deeper.

If there is a chemical in the eye:
   a. Call 9-1-1 or the local emergency number.
   b. Hold the injured eye open.
   c. Turn the athlete's head to the side so that the injured eye is below the uninjured eye. In this position, water can be used to flush the chemical away from the unaffected eye.
   d. Flush the injured eye with warm water for 15 to 20 continuous minutes.

TIP

Do not use chemical ice packs near a victim's eyes; use actual ice. Chemical ice packs could leak and burn the eyes.

Mouth Injuries

Many injuries to the mouth can be prevented through use of a mouth guard. In contact sports, athletes should wear mouth guards not only for competitions, but also for practices.

To care for an athlete with a knocked-out tooth:

1. Stop the bleeding by placing a rolled gauze pad in the empty tooth socket and directing the athlete to bite down.
2. Save the tooth by either:
   a. Rinsing the tooth gently and inserting it back into the tooth socket so that the top is even with the other teeth (if more than 30 minutes from a dentist and can do this without difficulty or causing further pain).
   b. Preserving the tooth in a container of saliva or milk (and bring the athlete to the dentist to reimplant the tooth).
3. If the tooth is fractured, be sure to try to find the missing segment and bring it to the dentist.
4. If an athlete has suffered an intrusion (the tooth is pushed up into the gums), use ice, control the bleeding, and see a dentist within 24 hours.

CAUTION

DO NOT put the tooth in mouthwash, alcohol, or water.

DO NOT remove partly knocked-out teeth.

DO NOT place a tooth back in the mouth of an unresponsive athlete because it may block the airway.

Nose Injuries

To care for an athlete with a nosebleed:

1. Have the athlete sit, lean slightly forward, and breathe through the mouth.
2. Pinch both nostrils steadily for 5 to 10 minutes

CAUTION

In controlling a nosebleed, DO NOT release the pressure prematurely to check if bleeding has stopped.

3. If bleeding continues, have the athlete gently sniff or blow their nose and pinch again for 5 to 10 minutes.
4. If bleeding still continues, seek medical care.
5. Discourage the athlete from swallowing blood.

To care for an athlete whose nose looks crooked after being hit:

1. Have the athlete sit, lean slightly forward, and breathe through the mouth.
2. Control any bleeding as just described.
3. Apply an ice pack to the nose for 20 minutes to reduce swelling and pain.
4. Seek medical care.

TIP

Helmet Removal Guidelines

Many injured athletes are wearing a helmet. Typically, helmets used by young athletes also have face shields, visors, or cages. It is very rare that a helmet would need to be removed from an injured athlete. The only instances when a helmet should be removed is if the helmet is interfering with the victim's breathing, if access to a nonbreathing athlete's airway is blocked, or if the helmet is so loose that adequate manual spinal stabilization cannot be provided. If the airway must be accessed, remove the face shield, visor, or cage while keeping the helmet in place. Most masks, visors, and cages are attached to helmets with a few screws. Removal of the screws (while maintaining manual spinal stabilization) usually allows for easy removal of the device. If it is absolutely necessary to remove the athlete's helmet, remove the shoulder pads as well to keep the spine aligned. It is imperative to maintain spinal stabilization during and after removal of the helmet. If the chin strap is not interfering, leave it in place. As a coach, be familiar with helmet construction and the methods of removing the face shield from the helmet. In most cases, it is best to await EMS arrival prior to removing the helmet.

Take this opportunity to locate a helmet. Find the appropriate tools and remove the face shield or visor from the helmet. Take note of the tools used; these tools should be available in the first-aid kit or at the sideline. If the shields cannot be removed, contact the manufacturer for instructions.

Spine Injuries

The spinal column consists of moveable vertebrae stacked from the tailbone to the base of the skull 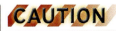. The *spinal column* is a complex network of bone (vertebrae), soft tissue (disks, muscles, and ligaments), joints, and nerves that can sustain injury during activity and athletic participation. The spinal cord and spinal nerves run throughout the spinal column and are the main communication network between the brain and the body. A fracture or dislocation of spinal vertebrae can potentially compress or cut the spinal cord or nerves and result in a permanent nonrecoverable injury.

Although serious spinal injuries are not common, a spinal cord or nerve injury could have lifelong devastating consequences. Depending on the spinal level involved in the injury, spinal cord injuries could result in muscle paralysis or affect vital life functions such as breathing. Less serious injuries such as sprains and strains are more common and should be treated like any other sprains or strains.

All unresponsive injury victims should be treated as though they have a serious spinal injury. All responsive victims sustaining injuries from falls, collisions with other players or the ground, or trauma that forces bending of the head or neck in any direction or produces a head injury, should be carefully checked prior to being moved.

CAUTION

Suspect a spinal injury in all head injury victims.

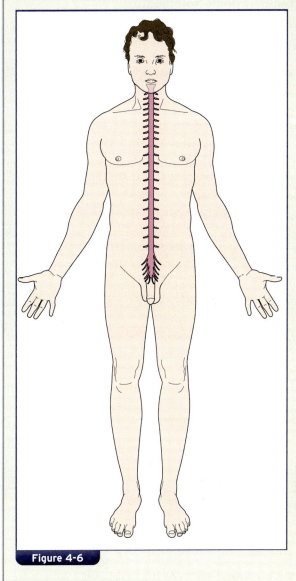

Figure 4-6

The spine contains bone, soft tissue, joints, and nerves that can be injured during athletic activity.

An athlete with a serious spinal injury may have any of the following:

- Neck or back pain
- Heaviness, weakness, burning, tingling, or loss of sensation in the arms or legs
- Loss of bowel or bladder control
- Paralysis of the arms or legs

To care for an athlete with a suspected spinal injury:

1. **Do not move the victim.**
2. Stabilize the spine. Use the manual spinal stabilization technique until trained personnel arrive with the proper equipment to stabilize the spine.
3. Do not remove the helmet unless the airway is compromised.
4. Monitor breathing. Perform CPR skills as indicated.
5. Call 9-1-1 or the local emergency number.

Manual Spinal Stabilization

Immediate stabilization of a victim with a suspected spinal injury is one of the most critical actions one can take in preventing a permanent spinal injury. EMS providers use specialized long spine boards, cervical collars, and sophisticated neck stabilization devices to stabilize the spine in victims with suspected spinal injuries. Most coaches neither have access to this equipment nor are trained in its use. A modified technique called *manual spinal stabilization* can be used to stabilize the spine until additional help arrives.

To provide manual spinal stabilization:

1. Instruct the alert victim not to move. Explain what is being done.
2. Be sure no one else attempts to move or excessively manipulate the victim.
3. The victim should remain flat on his or her back.
4. The person who will be providing the manual spinal stabilization should position him- or herself at the victim's head. They should gently but firmly secure the head around the ears to prevent any movement of the head or neck **Figure 4-7**. The helmet should be left on unless the victim's airway is compromised.

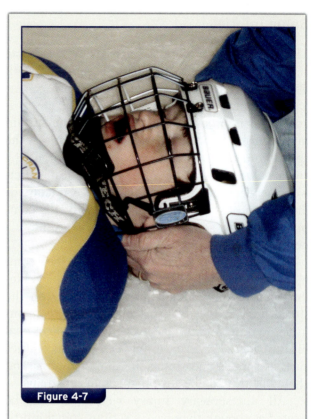

Figure 4-7

Secure the head around the ears to prevent movement of the head or neck.

CAUTION

DO NOT move an athlete with a suspected spinal injury until EMS arrives.

Chest Injuries

An athlete may sustain chest trauma resulting in bruising, fractured ribs, or a sprained/strained rib cage **Figure 4-8**. It should be noted that localized trauma to the breast bone (such as a direct blow to the chest) can result in serious internal injuries. If a direct blow to the chest is sustained, be sure to maintain a high index of suspicion for serious injury and seek appropriate care as soon as possible. Any unexplained chest pain or tightness in an athlete should be treated as a medical condition until proven otherwise. To care for an athlete with a chest injury:

1. Remove the athlete from competition.
2. Apply ice to the area for 20 minutes.
3. If the athlete experiences unresponsiveness, shortness of breath, or other serious symptoms, seek immediate medical care.
4. Require doctor clearance prior to return to play if pain or swelling persists.

Although rare, serious complications secondary to blunt chest trauma could have serious consequences in the athlete. Two such conditions are commotio cordis and cardiac contusion. *Commotio cordis* affects the heart and can occur when a blunt object such as a baseball (most common), a hockey puck, or any hard object strikes the chest at a particular moment in the cardiac cycle, causing sudden cardiac arrest. Most believe an undetected cardiac abnormality increases an athlete's risk of this condition. This can be prevented by wearing the proper equipment, such as a chest protector, which disperses the force across the entire chest. *Cardiac con-*

TIP

If a penetrating chest injury is present, secure the object with bulky dressings and prevent air leakage from the chest cavity by using an occlusive dressing such as Vaseline gauze or aluminum foil. Never remove a penetrating object from the chest.

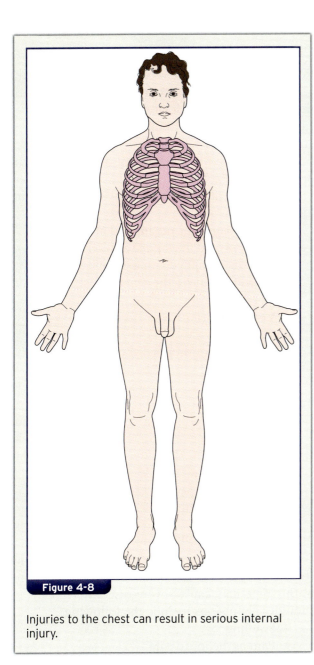

Figure 4-8

Injuries to the chest can result in serious internal injury.

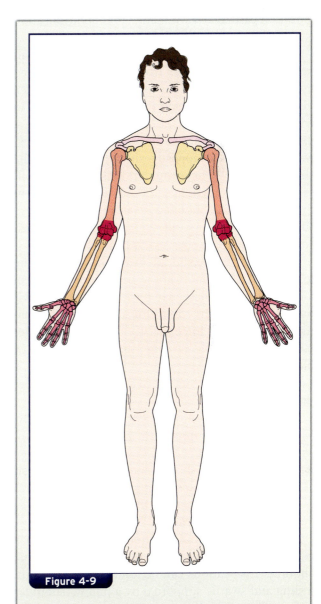

Figure 4-9

The upper extremity includes the area from the collarbone down through the fingertips.

tusion may occur when a blunt force to the chest causes bruising or swelling of tissues in the heart, which results in muscle death, a process similar to a heart attack. Make sure the athlete's equipment fits and support efforts to have an AED on the sideline.

Upper Extremity Injuries

Athletes in a variety of sports may sustain injuries to the shoulder, collarbone, arm, elbow, wrist, or fingers **Figure 4-9** .

Shoulder Dislocation

Three bones come together at the shoulder: the *scapula* (shoulder blade), the *clavicle* (collarbone), and the *humerus* (upper arm bone). The shoulder is the most freely movable joint in the body. The extreme range of its possible movements makes the shoulder joint highly susceptible to *dislocation* (separation). A dislocation of the shoulder occurs when the bones of the shoulder come apart as a result of a blow or a particular movement. Shoulder dislocation is second in frequency only to finger dislocation.

Many victims of a shoulder dislocation will hold the upper arm away from the body, supported by the uninjured arm. This position differentiates a dislocation from a fracture of the humerus, in which the victim holds the arm against the chest. A dislocated arm cannot be brought across the chest wall to touch the opposite shoulder (that is, the sling position). The shoulder looks squared off, rather than rounded, and there is extreme pain in the shoulder area. Shoulder dislocation also may result in numbness or paralysis in the arm from pressure and pinched blood vessels or nerves.

An injury to the shoulder resulting in complete loss of function is more apt to be a dislocation than a fracture. The athlete may have a history of previous dislocations. In caring for a shoulder dislocation, do not try to force, twist, or pull the shoulder back in place because it may cause bone, nerve, or blood vessel injury.

To care for an athlete with a suspected shoulder dislocation:

1. Place a folded or rolled blanket or a pillow between the upper arm and the chest to support the arm.
2. Stabilize the shoulder in a comfortable position or apply a sling and swathe.
3. Apply an ice pack to the painful area.
4. Seek medical care.

A dislocated shoulder should be splinted in a position most comfortable for the victim. Most shoulder dislocations can be safely immobilized in a sling and swathe supported by a pillow (shoulder sling and swathe). If the arm is hanging to the side, the use of one or two swathes to secure the arm to the victim's torso is adequate.

Clavicle Fracture

Fractures of the *clavicle* (collarbone) are common. Most clavicle fractures occur in the middle third of the bone. Usually the fracture is easy to detect because the clavicle lies immediately under the skin and a deformity can be seen. The victim of a fractured collarbone likely fell on an outstretched arm or received a direct blow to the clavicle or shoulder.

Symptoms of a fractured clavicle include the following:

- Severe pain over the injured area
- Desire to hold the injured arm against the chest with the uninjured arm to stabilize the injury
- Inability to move the arm because of the pain
- Swelling
- Visible deformity
- Tenderness
- "Dropped" or drooped shoulder
- Bruising

Take the following steps in caring for a clavicle fracture:

1. Place the victim in a comfortable position, such as sitting or lying flat on his or her back.
2. Apply an arm sling and swathe to immobilize the arm **Skill Drill 4-1** .
3. Apply an ice pack to the area.
4. Seek immediate medical care.

Shoulder Contusions

Direct blows to the shoulder can cause contusions (bruises). Often called *shoulder pointers*, contusions of this type may cause severe discomfort. Signs of shoulder contusions include the following:

- Swelling
- Pain at the injury site
- Feeling of firmness when pressure is exerted on the shoulder
- Tenderness
- Discoloration under the skin (black and blue)

To care for shoulder contusions:

1. Apply an ice pack to the area for 20 minutes, three to four times during the first 24 hours.
2. A sling and swathe or commercially available sling can be used to rest the arm.
3. Seek medical care if no improvement is noted within 24 hours.

skill drill

4-1 Sling for Clavicle or Shoulder Injury

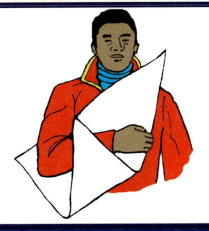

1 Place the bandage between the forearm and chest with its point toward the elbow and stretching beyond it. Pull the upper end over the shoulder on the uninjured side. Bring the other end of the bandage over the forearm and tuck it under the armpit on the injured side.

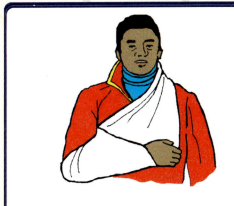

2 Continue bringing the lower end of the bandage around the victim's back where it is tied to the upper end of the bandage.

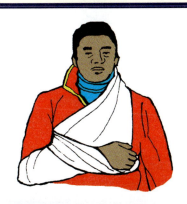

3 Place a swathe around the chest and forearm rather than the upper arm. The center of the swathe should be placed over the forearm. The hand should be in a thumb-up position within the sling and slightly above the level of the elbow.

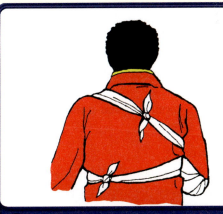

4 Tie the swathe behind the victim's back.

Tendinitis in the Shoulder Area

Tendinitis occurs when the tendons in and around the shoulder become inflamed. Occasionally, tendinitis may be accompanied by inflammation of the bursa sacs as well. Tendinitis is most commonly caused by overuse or unusual use. Tendinitis of the shoulder is most commonly seen in athletes involved in throwing (such as a baseball pitcher or a football quarterback) and in other sports in which the shoulder is used extensively (such as tennis and swimming).

Symptoms of tendinitis include:

- Constant pain or pain with motion of the shoulder
- Limited motion of the shoulder
- Cracking sound when the joint is moved
- Tenderness over the inflamed area
- Pain in the upper front part of the arm (biceps area)

Use the following steps to care for an athlete with these symptoms:

1. Restrict or reduce the activity for several days.
2. Correct any poor or improper mechanics during the motion.
3. Be sure the athlete warms up properly and is not overusing the shoulder.
4. Use ice for 20 minutes after the activity.
5. Any prolonged shoulder pain needs a consultation with a doctor or practitioner familiar with sports injuries.
6. A doctor may recommend ice massage for 10 minutes after exercise.
7. A doctor may recommend anti-inflammatory or pain medication.

Upper Arm Fracture

The humerus commonly is fractured when an athlete receives a direct blow to the upper arm or twists and falls on an outstretched arm.

- Symptoms include severe pain, swelling, tenderness, and visible deformity.
- The deformity may be hidden by swelling or by the large muscles surrounding the upper part of the arm.
- The athlete may be unable to move the arm and will hold the arm against the chest for comfort.

The following steps should be used when caring for an athlete with a humerus fracture.

1. Place the athlete in a comfortable position (sitting or lying flat on back).
2. Apply an ice pack.
3. Stabilize the arm by applying a rigid splint on the outer part of the arm away from the body **Figure 4-10**.
4. Apply an arm sling and swathe **Skill Drill 4-2**.
5. Seek immediate medical care.

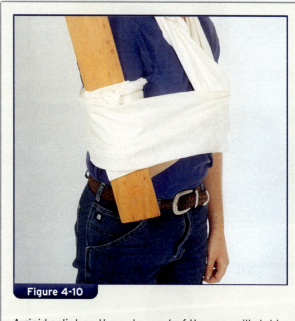

Figure 4-10

A rigid splint on the outer part of the arm will stabilize it.

TIP

Improvised Slings

If bandages or other resources are unavailable, you may need to improvise a sling **Figure 4-11**.

Elbow Fractures and Dislocations

All elbow fractures and dislocations should be considered serious and treated with extreme care. Inappropriate care can result in injury to the nearby

skill drill

4-2   Sling for Arm Injury

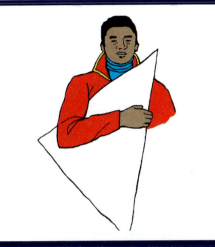

1 Place the bandage between the forearm and chest with the point of the bandage toward the elbow and stretch beyond the elbow. Pull the upper end of the bandage over the uninjured shoulder.

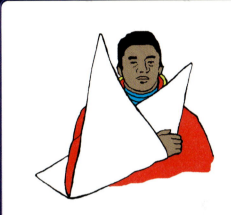

2 Bring the lower end of the bandage over the forearm.

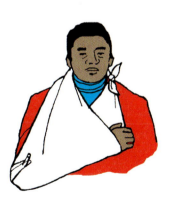

3 Bring the end of the bandage around the neck to the uninjured side and tie it to the other end at the hollow above the clavicle on the uninjured side.

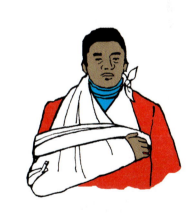

4 Place a swathe around the upper arm and body. The center of the swathe should be placed over the arm. The hand should be in thumb-up position within the sling and slightly above the level of the elbow.

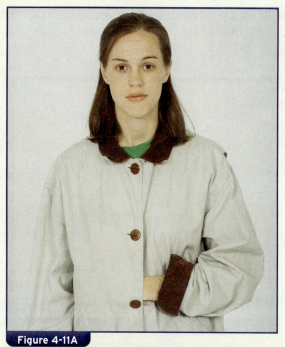

Figure 4-11A

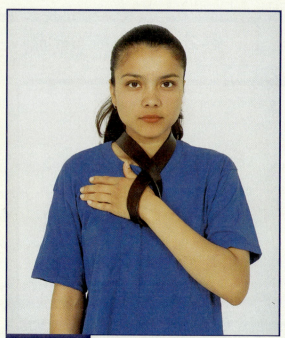

Figure 4-11B

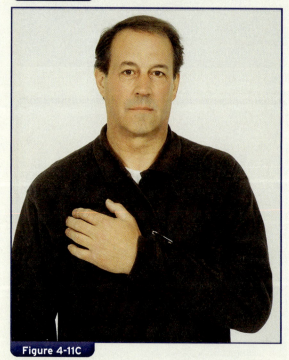

Figure 4-11C

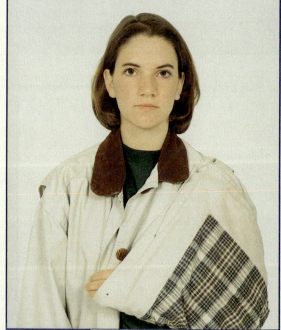

Figure 4-11D

Improvised slings. **A.** A buttoned jacket. **B.** A belt, necktie, or other clothing item looped around the neck and the injured arm. **C.** Sleeve of the jacket or shirt pinned to the clothing. **D.** Lower edge of the victim's jacket or shirt pinned up over the injured arm.

nerves and blood vessels. Symptoms of elbow fractures and dislocations include:

- Immediate swelling, severe pain, possible visible deformity (compared to the uninjured elbow)
- Restricted and painful motion
- Numbness or coldness of the hand and fingers below the elbow

To care for a suspected elbow fracture or dislocation:

1. Do not move the elbow.
2. Place the athlete in a comfortable position (sitting or lying on back).
3. Splint the elbow in the position found to prevent nerve and blood vessel damage **Figure 4-12** :

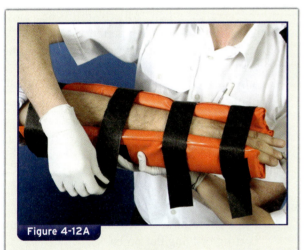

Figure 4-12A

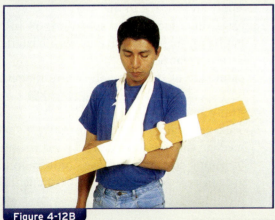

Figure 4-12B

A. If the elbow is straight, splint it straight. **B.** If the elbow is bent, splint it bent.

- If straight, splint the elbow straight.
- If bent, splint the elbow bent.

4. Apply an ice pack.
5. Seek immediate medical care.

Tennis Elbow

Tennis elbow can result from any activity that requires quick repetitive twists of the forearm (not just from playing tennis). The muscles and tendons that bend the wrist back and straighten the fingers attach to a small prominence on the outside of the elbow. Symptoms of tennis elbow result when these tendons become inflamed.

Consider tennis elbow if:

- The pain increases while using the arm or causes a gradual grip weakness.
- The injured elbow fatigues quicker than normal.
- The elbow is very tender on its outer protrusion.

Use the following steps to care for an athlete with these symptoms:

1. Restrict or reduce painful activities for several days.
2. Correct any poor or improper mechanics during the motion.
3. Be sure the athlete warms up properly and is not overusing the arm.
4. Use ice for 20 minutes after the activity.
5. Any prolonged shoulder pain needs a consultation with a doctor or practitioner familiar with sports injuries.
6. A doctor may recommend ice massage for 10 minutes after exercise.
7. A doctor may recommend anti-inflammatory or pain medication.

Little League or Golfer's Elbow

The conditions of Little League or golfer's elbow are the equivalent of the more common tennis elbow but with pain on the inside of the elbow. It is tendinitis affecting the tendons attached to the bony protrusion on the inside of the elbow.

Little League or golfer's elbow can be recognized when:

- Pain increases while using the arm.
- The athlete reports gradual weakness in the grip.

TIP

If a young athlete, especially a baseball pitcher, complains of pain on the inner protrusion of the elbow, he or she should be evaluated by a health care provider as soon as possible to rule out injury to the growth plate. In young baseball pitchers, proper warm-up, a plan to slowly increase pitch count, and strict attention to technique can help prevent Little League elbow.

- The injured elbow fatigues quicker than normal.
- The elbow is very tender on its inner protrusion.

Use the following steps to care for an athlete with these symptoms:

1. Restrict or reduce the activity for several days.
2. Correct any poor or improper mechanics during the motion.
3. Be sure the athlete warms up properly and is not overusing the elbow or arm.
4. Use ice for 20 minutes after the activity.
5. Any prolonged shoulder pain needs a consultation with a doctor or practitioner familiar with sports injuries.
6. A doctor may recommend ice massage for 10 minutes after exercise.
7. A doctor may recommend anti-inflammatory or pain medication.

Radius and Ulna Fractures

There are two large bones in the forearm, the radius and the ulna, and either or both of these bones may be broken. When only one bone is fractured, the other bone acts as a splint. In this case, there may be little or no deformity. However, a marked deformity may be present in fractures near the wrist. When both bones are broken, the arm usually appears deformed.

A radius or ulna fracture should be suspected if the athlete has pain in the forearm or wrist from a direct blow or falling on an outstretched hand. The athlete may have:

- A visible deformity
- Severe pain radiating up and down from the injury site

- An inability to move the wrist or pain while moving the wrist or elbow

An athlete with a forearm fracture requires the following care:

1. Place the athlete in a comfortable position (sitting or lying flat on back).
2. Apply an ice pack to the area.
3. Apply two rigid splints on both sides of the arm from the tip of the elbow to the fingers. Place the arm in an arm sling and swathe.
4. Seek medical care.

Wrist Fracture

The wrist usually is broken when the victim falls on the arm with the hand outstretched. Wrist fractures are common in victims who fall backwards and try to break their fall with an outstretched arm (such as falling backwards when rollerblading or snow boarding). The athlete may experience:

- A snapping or popping sensation within the wrist
- Pain in the wrist that is aggravated by movement
- Tenderness and swelling
- Inability or unwillingness to move the wrist
- A lump-like deformity on the back of the wrist

An athlete with a wrist fracture requires the following care:

1. Place the athlete in a comfortable position (sitting or lying flat on back).
2. Apply an ice pack to the area.
3. Have the athlete grasp something in his or her hand, such as a rolled up elastic bandage or roller gauze. Place a rigid splint on the palm side of the arm and secure the splint with an elastic bandage **Figure 4-13**.
4. Apply an arm sling and swathe.
5. Seek medical care. It is imperative to seek medical care for all suspected wrist fractures in young athletes because injuries to the growth areas could result in permanent deformities.

Finger Fracture

Contrary to popular belief, broken bones—especially the fingers—may be able to move when they are broken. The athlete may have:

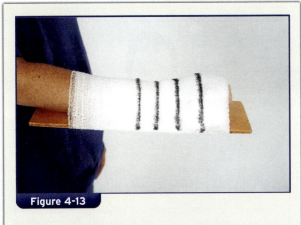

Figure 4-13

Place a rigid splint on the palm side of the arm and secure the splint with a roller bandage.

- A visible deformity; the finger has a twisted look
- Immediate localized pinpoint pain
- Pain with or without movement
- Numbness
- Swelling

In caring for finger fractures:

1. Do not try to realign the finger.
2. Gently apply an ice pack.
3. Splint the finger by buddy taping the fractured finger to another for support **Figure 4-14**.
4. Seek medical care for all finger fractures in young athletes because injuries to the growth areas could result in permanent deformities.

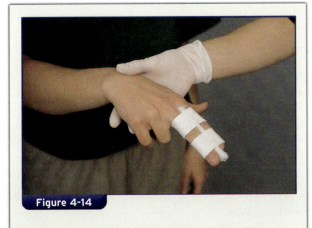

Figure 4-14

Use of a buddy splint is recommended for fractured fingers.

Finger Dislocation

Finger dislocations are common. The same causes of fractured fingers also can cause a dislocated finger. Indications of a finger dislocation include:

- A visible deformity in the finger or thumb
- Immediate pain, swelling, and shortening of the finger
- An athlete's inability to bend the finger in the injured area

In caring for an athlete with a finger dislocation:

1. Do not try to realign the dislocation.
2. Apply an ice pack.
3. If possible, splint the finger by buddy taping it to another finger.
4. Seek medical care.

Sprained Finger

Several ligaments surround each joint in the fingers. Athletes with a sprained finger usually report that the finger was "jammed" or compressed, stepped on, or forced or twisted sideways. There are three joints in each finger and two in each thumb; any of these joints can be injured.

An athlete with a sprained finger likely has:

- Pain and swelling over one or several finger joints
- Inability to make a fist
- Weakness while curling the injured finger alone
- Weakness or pain when gripping

Follow these steps in caring for a sprained finger:

1. Apply an ice pack for 20 minutes.
2. Use buddy taping for support.
3. Seek medical care if pain persists. Remember, only an x-ray can rule out a fracture.

Nail Avulsion

A nail avulsion victim may have had a blow to the fingernail or the nail may have been torn away by a piece of equipment. An injury in which a nail is partly or completely torn loose is known as a *nail avulsion*. Take the following steps to care for a nail avulsion:

- Secure the damaged nail in place with an adhesive bandage or tape.
- If part or the entire nail has been completely torn away:

- Apply antibiotic ointment.
- Secure the loose nail with an adhesive bandage or tape.
- Do not trim away the loose nail.
- Consult a doctor for further advice.

Splinters

Sharp splinters can be impaled into the skin or under a fingernail or toenail. There is a small puncture wound and the sliver may or may not be seen or felt. If a splinter is embedded in the skin:

- Use tweezers to remove it.
- In some cases, it may be possible to "tease" it out with a sterile needle until the end can be grasped with tweezers or fingers.
- Clean the wound with soap and water.
- Apply an antibiotic ointment.
- Seek medical care if signs of infection occur.
- If the splinter is impaled under a fingernail or toenail and breaks off, seek medical care.

Blood Under a Nail

Blood collects under a fingernail when underlying tissues are bruised. Excruciating pain exists because of the pressure of the blood pushing against the nail. Pain does not disappear until the collection of blood is drained.

Take the following steps in caring for blood under a nail:

1. Immerse the finger in ice water or apply an ice pack.
2. Elevate to reduce pain and swelling.
3. Seek medical care as soon as possible to drain the fluid from under the nail.

Lower Extremity Injuries

The lower extremities include the hip, upper leg, knee, lower leg, ankle, foot, and toes **Figure 4-15**.

Hip Dislocation

A hip can be dislocated by a fall, a blow to the thigh, or direct force to the foot or knee. The hip joint is a stable ball-and-socket joint that requires great force to dislocate. It is difficult to differentiate a hip dislocation from a hip fracture. An athlete with a hip dislocation has:

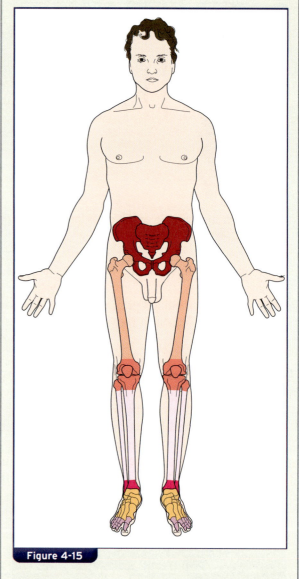

Figure 4-15

The lower extremity includes the area from the hip down through the toes.

- Severe pain and/or swelling at the injury site
- A flexed hip and the knee bent and rotated inward toward the opposite hip
- Deformity in the hip area

An athlete with a hip dislocation requires the following care:

1. Place the athlete lying flat on his or her back.

2. Call 9-1-1 or the local emergency number.
3. Apply an ice pack to the area.
4. Attempt to immobilize the area for minimal movement.
5. Buddy taping the leg on the injured side to the uninjured side may help reduce pain **Figure 4-16**. Do this only if EMS is delayed.
6. Be aware of other injuries including a spinal injury.

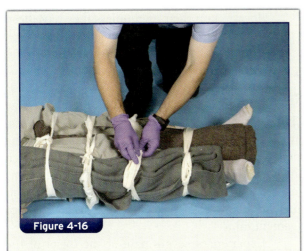

Figure 4-16

Putting the injured leg in a buddy splint may help reduce pain.

Hip Fracture

A hip fracture is a fracture of the upper end of the *femur* (thighbone). An athlete with a hip fracture has:

- Severe pain in the groin area
- Inability to lift the injured leg
- Apparent shortened leg, which may be rotated with the toes pointing abnormally outward

An athlete with a hip fracture requires the following care:

1. Place the athlete lying flat on his or her back.
2. Call 9-1-1 or the local emergency number.
3. Apply an ice pack to the injured area.
4. Attempt to stabilize the area for minimal movement.

5. Buddy taping the leg on the injured side to the uninjured side may help reduce pain. Do this only if EMS is delayed.
6. Be aware of other injuries to the victim, including spinal injuries.

Thigh Injuries

Because the femur is the largest bone in the body, considerable force is required to break it. Femur injuries can occur in any part of the femur, from the hip area to just above the knee joint. A fracture of the femur usually is caused by a fall or a direct blow. Femur fractures may include open wounds and external bleeding may be severe. If the blood vessels are damaged and internal bleeding occurs within the thigh, the victim could lose 1 or 2 quarts of blood. There may be loss of blood circulation to the lower part of the extremity or nerve damage, especially when the lower third of the femur is fractured. The following signs and symptoms may indicate a femur fracture:

- Severe pain at the injury site
- Deformity—the leg may appear shorter
- Swelling from severe damage to blood vessels
- Victim heard or felt a severe pop or snap at the time of injury

An athlete with a suspected femur fracture requires the following care:

1. Place the athlete lying flat on his or her back.
2. Call 9-1-1 or the local emergency number.
3. Apply an ice pack to the injured area.
4. Attempt to immobilize the area for minimal movement.
5. Buddy taping the leg on the injured side to the uninjured side may help reduce pain. Do this only if EMS is delayed.
6. Be aware of other injuries to the victim including spinal injury.

Muscle Contusion

The muscle group on the front of the thigh is the quadriceps group and often gets bruised. Depending on the force of impact and the muscles involved, the contusion may be of varying degrees of severity. Suspect a muscle contusion if the victim received a direct hit and is experiencing the following symptoms:

- Swelling, pain, and tenderness
- Tightness or firmness
- Visible bruise (may appear hours later)

In caring for an athlete with a muscle contusion:

1. Stop the activity.
2. Apply an ice pack for 20 minutes, three to four times daily for the next 48 hours.
3. If not improving, seek medical care.

Knee Fractures

A fracture of the knee generally occurs as a result of a fall or a direct blow. Fractures about the knee may occur at the end of the femur, at the end of the *tibia* (lower leg), or in the *patella* (kneecap). Determining if a fracture exists is difficult. Some fractured knees may look like a dislocation. Other signs include the following:

- Deformity
- Tenderness
- Swelling, which may be perceived by the athlete as fullness in the back of the knee above the calf

Care for suspected knee fractures as follows:

1. Stabilize the leg in the found position.
2. Call 9-1-1 or the local emergency number.
3. Apply ice to the injured area.
4. Buddy taping the leg on the injured side to the uninjured side may help reduce pain.
5. In athletes, protective equipment may be used as a rigid splint.

Knee Dislocation

A knee dislocation is a serious injury. Deformity will be grotesque and the athlete will experience excruciating pain. Do not confuse a knee dislocation with a patella dislocation. A knee dislocation is a much more serious injury. It is important to stabilize the knee in the position found and to seek medical care immediately.

Kneecap Dislocation

A dislocated patella occurs when the kneecap becomes forcefully misaligned by either trauma or the twisting of the leg. It is common in young athletes. A dislocated patella usually is easily seen. An athlete with a possible kneecap dislocation may have:

- Pain in the area
- Swelling
- An inability to bend or straighten the knee.
- Deformity (compare it with the other kneecap). The kneecap is misaligned to either the inside or the outside of the knee joint.

To care for an athlete with a dislocated patella:

1. Stop the activity and have the athlete sit or lie down.
2. Apply ice.
3. Do not try to relocate a dislocated kneecap. Sometimes the kneecap replaces itself.
4. Discourage the athlete from relocating a dislocation on their own unless they have been directed to do so by a medical practitioner.
5. Stabilize the knee in the position found.
6. Seek medical care.

Knee Sprain

The knee has several ligaments for support. Excessive forces caused by external trauma; rapid, twisting movements; and missteps commonly overstretch and/or tear these ligaments. The external (*collateral*) and internal (*cruciate*) ligaments are commonly injured in athletes. An athlete with a suspected knee ligament injury:

- Experiences severe pain at the onset of the injury
- Reports feeling a pop or snap
- May have a locked knee or have the sensation of his or her knee locking
- May not be able to walk without limping
- May not be able to bend or straighten the knee
- May have swelling and bruising in the knee

To care for an athlete with a suspected knee ligament injury:

1. Stop the activity.
2. Have the athlete take all their weight off the injured knee.
3. Apply ice.
4. Apply a compression bandage.
5. Seek medical care.

Lower Leg Fractures

Fractures to the lower leg may affect the *tibia* (larger shin bone), the *fibula* (smaller bone on the outside of the lower leg), or both. A direct blow or twisting forces to the lower leg that produces severe pain, swelling, visible deformity, and tenderness suggests a possible fracture of one or both of these bones.

- When both bones are broken, there is a marked deformity of the leg.
- When only one bone is broken, the other may act as a splint, and little deformity may be present. Some victims with a fibula fracture can walk on the injured leg.

To care for a victim with a suspected lower leg fracture:

1. Place the athlete lying flat on his or her back.
2. Apply an ice pack to the area.
3. Apply a splint. Do your best to immobilize the area with minimal movement. Use a pillow splint **Figure 4-17**, especially if the suspected fracture is near the ankle.
4. Seek medical care.

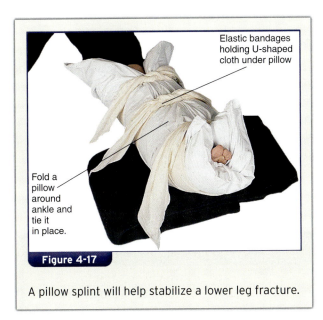

Elastic bandages holding U-shaped cloth under pillow

Fold a pillow around ankle and tie it in place.

Figure 4-17

A pillow splint will help stabilize a lower leg fracture.

Tibia and Fibula Contusion

Many contusions simply cause a black-and-blue mark and some soreness, and clear up with little attention. If an athlete received a contusion from a direct hit on the shin, the area will be tender when

touched and the athlete will feel a sharp pain. Later there will be:

- Discoloration (black-and-blue mark)
- Difficulty moving the ankle up and down
- Numbness or coldness in toes or foot

To care for a tibia or fibula contusion:

1. Stop the activity.
2. Use an ice pack for 20 minutes, three to four times daily for the first 48 hours.
3. If numbness or tingling exists beyond 24 hours, seek medical care.

Muscle Cramp

Muscle spasm or cramping usually occurs in the calf and sometimes in the thigh or hamstring. It is a temporary condition of little consequence. A muscle cramp often happens during or after intense exercise sessions. It causes a painful muscle contraction or spasm that may disable the athlete or may cause localized pain.

There are many treatments for muscle cramps. Try one or more of the following:

- Take all weight off the painful area.
- Have the victim gently stretch the affected muscle. Because a muscle cramp is an uncontrolled muscle contraction or spasm, a gradual extension of the muscle may help lengthen the muscle fibers and relieve the cramp.
- Relax the muscle by applying pressure to it.
- Apply heat.
- Pinch the upper lip hard (an acupressure technique) to reduce calf muscle cramping.
- Be sure the athlete is properly hydrated.

Shin Splints

The term *shin splints* is commonly used to describe pain in the front of the lower leg. Shin splints result when excessive stresses cause the tendon in the lower leg to pull from the bone. Shin splints usually are caused by repetitive stress in the leg, commonly resulting from a new activity or rapid increases in an existing activity. Shin splints are often the result of changes in workout routines, such as an increase in workout time or distance or changes in training terrain (eg, runners who add uphill running to their routines). The athlete may complain of:

- Pain during and immediately after the activity
- Pain alleviated with rest

The athlete may not want to train due to the pain or may frequently rest during activity. Athletes with suspected shin splints should be evaluated and treated by medical personnel trained in the management of sports injuries. Shin splints may become chronic and commonly need medical intervention and rest for complete resolution.

Take the following steps when caring for shin splints (or as advised by a doctor):

1. Warm the area prior to activity with moist heat.
2. Apply pressure with a 3-inch elastic bandage over the sorest point (start below the sore area and spiral wrap up and around the leg).
3. Apply an ice pack for 20 minutes after the activity or use ice massage.
4. Reduce the activity until the shin is pain free.
5. A doctor may prescribe an anti-inflammatory drug.

Ankle Injuries

Ankle injuries are one of the more common injuries seen in athletes. Most ankle injuries are sprains, but fractures could occur anywhere in the ankle area. The majority of ankle sprains involve the lateral (outside) ligaments and are caused by having the ankle turned or twisted inward. Whether an ankle is broken or sprained is difficult to assess without an x-ray. The Ottawa Ankle Rules (adapted in Table 4-2) can help determine if an ankle is fractured or sprained. This table is included for demonstration purposes, because use of these procedures is intended for trained medical personnel. When a coach suspects an ankle injury, medical consultation almost always is indicated. Prompt medical care and proper treatment results in faster recovery and return to play.

To care for an athlete with a suspected ankle sprain:

1. Stop the activity and take all weight off the injured ankle.
2. Apply ice to the area for 20 minutes, three to five times per day.
3. Elevate the injured ankle.
4. Apply a compression bandage.
5. If the injury appears severe, apply a pillow splint and seek medical care.
6. Seek medical care to ensure a proper rehabilitation program or to rule out a fracture.

Toe Injuries

The toes can be injured in a variety of ways. The toes can be stepped on or the foot may be kicked against a hard object, resulting in nail injuries, dislocations, or fractures. For nail avulsions, splinters, blood under a nail, dislocations, and fractures, refer to the appropriate sections under Finger Injuries.

Table 4-2 Ottawa Ankle Rules (Adapted)

If the Athlete:	
1. Cannot bear weight and take four steps immediately after the injury, and 2. Complains of tenderness at the back edge or tip of either ankle knob (the projections on each side of the ankle) when pressed	**Suspect a broken ankle.**
If the Athlete:	
1. Can bear weight and take four steps immediately after the injury, and 2. Does not complain about tenderness when the back edge or tip of either ankle knob is pressed	**Suspect a sprained ankle.**

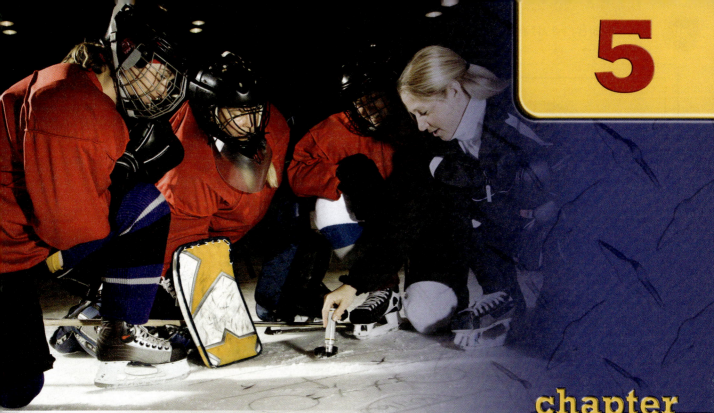

Phases of Injury: The Injury Prevention Model

chapter
at a glance

▶ **Introduction**

▶ **The Preinjury Phase**

▶ **The Injury Phase**

▶ **The Postinjury Phase**

▶ **Summary of the Injury Prevention Model**

▶ Introduction

Calling an injury an accident suggests that the injury was not preventable and that there was little that could be done to minimize the extent of the injury. Although rapid first aid can have a dramatic effect on an injured athlete, it must be appreciated that this effect is somewhat limited by the extent of the injury itself. An injury cannot be undone; however, strategies exist to prevent the injury from occurring and methods that limit or reduce the actual transmission of forces during the impact are just as important as high-quality first aid.

Those responsible for youth athletes—including team-governing bodies, parents, and coaches—must consider prevention strategies before the season begins. Coaches must assess every injury immediately after it occurs and review injury trends at the end of each season. In addition to managing injuries that do occur, coaches must carefully search for preventive strategies that reduce reoccurrence of injuries. One method that injury prevention specialists use to help reduce injury is the injury prevention model **Figure 5-1**. The injury prevention model examines three phases of injury control designed to reduce and control an injury before it occurs, as it is occurring, and after it

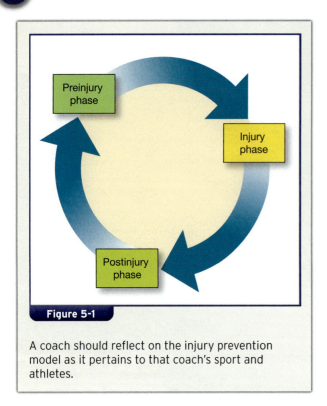

Figure 5-1

A coach should reflect on the injury prevention model as it pertains to that coach's sport and athletes.

has occurred (the focus of most first-aid programs). A coach should reflect frequently on the injury prevention model as it pertains to that coach's sport and athletes. The injury prevention model is divided into the preinjury phase, the injury phase, and the postinjury phase.

▶ The Preinjury Phase

The *preinjury phase* is a critical phase that occurs before the team places a foot on the playing field. If one were to scrutinize and trace the events that lead to an injury, it would not be surprising to locate a specific cause of the injury. Perhaps the injury was caused by a hole in the ground on a soccer field, a score table placed too close to the court, or an adolescent child wearing last season's equipment. The coach also may notice that many players are sustaining similar injuries stemming from a poor conditioning or training program.

The preinjury phase requires preparation and reflection of prevention strategies from numerous perspectives. Components of the preinjury phase include factors related to the athlete, the environment, the rules of the game, the officials and coaches, the medical team (if one exists), and the development of an emergency action plan (EAP). The following examples include strategies for a youth sport team.

The Athlete

- Is the athlete properly conditioned?
- Is the athlete's age, size, and skill level appropriate for the level of competition?
- Is the athlete wearing the proper equipment and does it all fit correctly? Is the equipment designed for the sport? Is a player wearing borrowed equipment because he or she forgot their own? Has equipment been modified? Is the athlete wearing last year's equipment? Is the athlete wearing the proper footwear for the surface and weather conditions?
- Does each athlete have his or her own water bottle? To prevent transmission of certain diseases, water bottles should not be shared among teammates.

TIP

Each player should have his or her own water bottle clearly labeled. This water bottle should be cleaned (or replaced) after each event.

The Environment

The environment includes areas used for practicing, warming up, and dressing (locker rooms). In smaller schools and gymnasiums, many athletes may warm up in a hallway, on a small auditorium stage, or in a small classroom.

- What is the condition of the playing surface? Consider weather, lighting, obstructions, hard or sharp surfaces, padded surfaces, open doors, and proximity of spectator seats to the playing surface.
- Where are the athletes warming up? Is the warm-up area safe? Is the warm-up area supervised?
- Is the locker room supervised? Are the showers safe? Are the locker rooms clean and properly disinfected?

The Rules of the Game

- Does everyone understand the rules of the game?

In The News

A young T-ball player was injured when the second baseman thought he had to throw the baseball at the player running the bases.

- Is everyone playing by the same rules?

In The News

A young girl sustained a broken nose in a tae kwon do competition when she was unaware that the rules had been changed to allow kicks to the head.

The Officials and Coaches

- Does the referee (especially at the youth levels) know the age range of the participants?

TIP

Prior to a game, it is useful to discuss the ages of the players on your team with the officials. In many sports, officials are paid to officiate several league/club games in a given time span, potentially creating confusion by the official during the actual competition.

- Does the coach have each player's medical history form? Is he or she aware of athletes with specific medical problems (eg, seizures, diabetes, or asthma)?
- Does the coach know where athletes' medications are located (inhaler, epinephrine autoinjector)? Are the medications clearly labeled with the athletes' names **Figure 5-2** ?
- Who is responsible for administering the medications? If a parent is not present, is the child capable of administering it to him- or herself? Does the coach have permission to administer it?
- Does the coach know the location and contents of the first-aid kit? Does the coach know how to use what is inside the first-aid kit?
- Are coaches and referees certified in coaching and first aid? Is there a certification program for a particular sport?
- Is there a league, organization, or other governing body that sets guidelines and standards for coaches?

The Medical Team

- Does a medical team exist for this event?
- Is there a sideline practitioner? What is his or her level of training: nurse, doctor, chiropractor, athletic trainer? What can they do and what are they prepared to do?
- Who will control bystanders such as anxious parents and others wanting to lend assistance

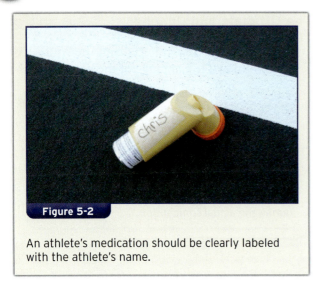

Figure 5-2

An athlete's medication should be clearly labeled with the athlete's name.

to the injured athlete? Are any of the parents health care providers? If so, are they adequately trained to deal with a sports injury?

- What does the medical team know about the sport? At higher levels of competition, there may be contracted emergency medical providers on the sidelines. Do coaches know where they are located? Do they have easy access to the playing field? Do they know when and how they will be notified to assist with the care of a patient?

In The News

An ambulance crew was booed by a high school football crowd due to an apparent slow response time. A review of the incident revealed that the athletic director parked in the ambulance parking space. The crew, not wanting to create trouble with the athletic director, parked the ambulance on the street near the main gate. They did not realize that the gate was blocked during the actual game; this significantly delayed their response time to the field.

Emergency Action Plan

An EAP should be created at the beginning of the season and modified on an ongoing basis (See Appendix A for a sample EAP form). It should be dis-

cussed with other coaches, parents, and club/team officials. The components of an EAP include the following:

- Who will attend to the sick or injured player? Is that person certified in CPR and first aid? Is there a trained back-up person if that person is not available?
- How will 9-1-1 be called in the event of an emergency (phone, radio)? Who will call 9-1-1 or any other emergency number?
- Who will stay (if necessary) with the sick or injured player when the competition resumes?
- Who will stay with the other players while the coach attends to the sick or injured?
- Where is the first-aid kit? What is in it?

TIP

Do not save opening your first-aid kit for the first injury of the season. Look inside, make sure it is stocked, and make sure you understand how to use the equipment and supplies in the kit.

- Is an AED available? If so, where?
- Who will be responsible for providing first aid if the coach is unavailable or not present?
- Are consent forms, medical history forms, and medication information readily available at all practices and competitions? What if the head coach cannot make a practice or game? Have the medical forms been turned over to the assistant coaching staff?
- What is the process for returning a player to play?

▶ The Injury Phase

Aside from being prepared for a potential injury and taking active steps to avoid the injury, there is little that can be done during the injury phase. This phase occurs at the moment of actual impact (or transmission of forces) and is greatly influenced by preinjury preparation. The major components of this phase include an athlete's injury threshold, his or her physical and mental conditioning, the athlete's attitude or mind-set, and the ability of the equipment to do what it was intended to do.

There is little a coach can do regarding an athlete's injury threshold besides properly training and conditioning the athlete. Whereas practice sessions should be designed to physically prepare an athlete for competition, good coaches also use practice time to mentally condition athletes for the upcoming competition. The mind-set of the athlete during this stage often can have an effect on the injury. Many coaches have experienced situations in which an injury has occurred secondary to a bad judgment made by a player. This could be retaliation against a prior "dirty" play or even the result of a bad call from an official. Such acts could be prevented by providing proper instruction of the rules of the game. Coaches can minimize an athlete's anxiety by showing restraint when responding to an official's call. Do not berate officials. Not only does this increase the coaches' and officials' anxiety, this also could increase the anxiety of the players and fans. At younger ages, this could potentially result in a bad judgment made by the athlete and subsequent harm to someone on the field.

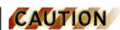

CAUTION

As a coach, watch your attitude during competition. Being hostile to the officials can lead to anxiety among players.

At the actual time of injury, the equipment must function and perform the action for which it was intended. It is not likely that equipment will ever be designed to offer 100% protection, but as technology and engineering concepts improve, equipment likely will become more protective. Although proper utilization of equipment is a preinjury consideration, the equipment's protective effect is valid only while the forces are being transmitted. For example, a helmet is useless to a player unless head impact occurs. Because the injury phase typically occurs in milliseconds, there is little a coach or first-aid provider can do beyond being properly prepared for this stage. They must ensure during the preinjury stage that all equipment is utilized, that it fits

properly, and that the best available technology is being used.

▶ The Postinjury Phase

Injury is a fact of sports participation and it is evident that preventing an injury is as important as treating an injury. Inevitably, even the most cautious coach will encounter an injured athlete at some point in his or her career. A well-prepared coach will take every step to ensure that preinjury and injury phase planning are properly executed. When an injury does occur, prompt management, follow-up, and analysis of the events that led to the injury are critical in reducing future injuries, as well as the loss of playing time and disability in their athletes.

The postinjury phase can be divided into three phases: the period immediately following the injury, the period between when an injury occurs and the time the athlete is released to a responsible adult or medical personnel, and the period between the athlete's release and when he or she returns to practice or competition.

Immediately Following an Injury

The period immediately following the injury is the time when good training in first aid is critical. Factors that come into play during this phase include:

- The coach's ability to identify injuries based on their unique knowledge of the athlete and the sport. For example, the coach is aware that one player has a history of asthma and now is lying on the court in apparent distress. The coach grabs the athlete's inhaler as he approaches the athlete.
- The coach's ability to control the situation (including noninjured players, coaches, trained and untrained bystanders, and multiple injuries).
- The coach's ability to provide evidence-based first-aid procedures (the performance of outdated and unsubstantiated actions by coaches, parents, and players should be discouraged).
- The coach's ability to know when additional help is needed and whether outside support (EMS) is required.

Between the Injury and Release

Actions to take in the period between the injury and the time the athlete is released to a responsible adult or medical personnel include:

- Identifying that an injured athlete needs additional medical care
- Conveying the extent of injuries and first aid provided to EMS or medical personnel
- Reevaluating an athlete who has sustained an injury
- Recognizing an injured athlete at the conclusion of the competition
- Releasing the athlete with instructions to care for and/or follow-up on an injury
- Ensuring that the athlete is released to a responsible adult

Before Return to Play

In the period between when the athlete leaves a coach's care and when he or she returns for the next session, critical actions include:

- Following up with an injured athlete (or parent) to ensure that the athlete received the proper care

- Determining when and if the player is ready to return to play
- Assessing the situation to determine if anything could be done to reduce the risk of a similar injury occurring in the future (Did the equipment do what it was supposed to do?)
- Maintaining and reviewing an injury log and taking the appropriate steps to minimize future injuries

▶ Summary of the Injury Prevention Model

An injury prevention program is multifaceted. An effective injury prevention program results from changes in knowledge, attitude, and behavior of coaches, athletes, league administrators, officials, and parents. Proper attention to all three phases of the injury prevention model minimizes an athlete's risk of injury, may help reduce the extent of an injury, and ensures a consistent and uniform approach for a safe and fun environment for a team.

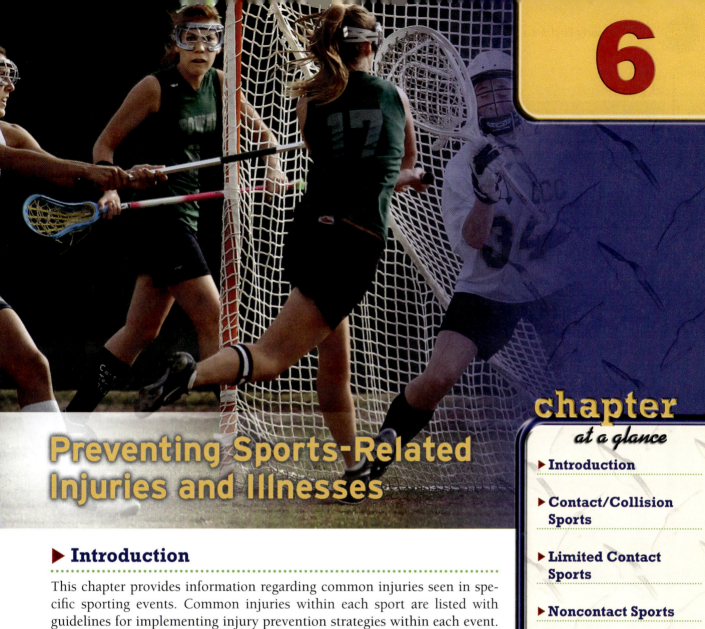

Preventing Sports-Related Injuries and Illnesses

chapter *at a glance*

▶ **Introduction**

▶ **Contact/Collision Sports**

▶ **Limited Contact Sports**

▶ **Noncontact Sports**

▶ Introduction

This chapter provides information regarding common injuries seen in specific sporting events. Common injuries within each sport are listed with guidelines for implementing injury prevention strategies within each event. It is worthwhile to review all the listed sports, even the ones with which a coach is not involved, because he or she may find useful ideas that can be modified for their sport.

Sporting events can be classified into collision contact, limited contact, and noncontact sports. **Table 6-1** categorizes a variety of sports into these classifications. Although injuries may occur in any sport, certain injuries such as head and spinal injuries are more common in collision contact sports. Categorizing a sport as a limited or noncontact sport does not, however, preclude the possibility of serious injuries. In many cases, limited and noncontact sports have incidental contact, which in the absence of protective equipment can have serious consequences.

Regardless of the classification level of a sport, coaches should strongly encourage participants to stay hydrated at all times during practice and com-

TIP

Review injuries, areas injured, and prevention guidelines for all sports, not just the ones you coach.

CAUTION

Even noncontact sports may have incidental contact, which in the absence of protective equipment can have serious consequences.

petition 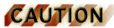 because heat-related injuries always are a potential threat. In addition, it is critical that coaches, parents, and fellow athletes deem-

phasize diet as a factor in body weight, physical appearance, and performance. Instead, good dietary habits, such as the avoidance of junk foods, foods

Table 6-1 Classification of Sports by Contact

Contact/Collision	Limited Contact	Noncontact
Basketball*	Baseball*	Archery
Boxing	Bicycling	Badminton
Diving	Canoeing/kayaking (white water)	Body building
Field hockey	Cheerleading*	Bowling
Football*	Fencing	Canoeing/kayaking (flat water)
Flag	Field*	Crew/rowing
Tackle*	High jump	Curling
Ice hockey*	Pole vault	Dancing
Lacrosse*	Floor hockey	Field*
Martial arts*	Gymnastics*	Discus
Rodeo	Handball	Javelin
Roller hockey*	Horseback riding	Shot put
Rugby	Racquetball	Golf
Ski jumping	Skating	Orienteering
Soccer*	Ice	Power lifting*
Team handball	Inline	Race walking
Water polo	Roller	Riflery
Wrestling*	Skiing	Rope jumping
	Cross-country	Running
	Downhill*	Sailing
	Water	Scuba diving
	Softball*	Strength training
	Squash	Swimming*
	Ultimate Frisbee	Table tennis
	Volleyball*	Tennis*
	Windsurfing/surfing	Track*
		Weight lifting*

*Sports included in this section
Source: Reproduced with permission from Pediatrics, Vol. 94, page 757, © 1994 by the AAP.

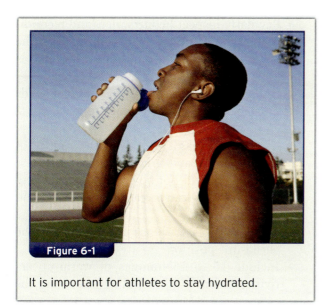

Figure 6-1

It is important for athletes to stay hydrated.

high in fat content, and carbonated beverages should be encouraged and facilitated.

Immediately remove from participation any athlete who sustains an open wound. The wound must be cleaned and covered with a protective dressing. Bleeding must be controlled before the athlete returns to participation. Bloody uniforms must be changed prior to return to participation. Coaches should always have appropriate first aid materials including protective gloves, sterile gauze pads (preferably 2" × 2" or larger), and bandages (elastic adhesive tape and/or elastic wraps) for controlling bleeding at all games and practices.

▶ Contact/Collision Sports

Basketball

Participation in basketball, regardless of age or level of play, often involves contact between players, and in some cases, collisions with another player can result in injuries ranging from minor to severe, depending on the body area(s) involved.

Most Common Basketball Injuries

- Sprains (joint injuries)
- Strains (muscle and tendon injuries)
- Contusions (bruises)

Body Areas Injured in Basketball

- Ankle and foot
- Hip, thigh, and leg
- Knee
- Forearm, wrist, and hand
- Face, scalp, and mouth (dental)

A major ligament of the knee known as the *anterior cruciate ligament (ACL)* is injured significantly more often in females than in males in basketball. Numerous theories have been proposed to explain this difference; however, no one theory has yet received majority approval from the sports medicine community. Research is ongoing, however, and presently many in the sports medicine community advise teaching young athletes to run and jump correctly, emphasizing good joint alignment in the lower extremities, and maintaining muscle strength in their hips, thighs, and lower legs.

Injury Prevention Guidelines for Basketball

- Coaches should be required to have current first aid and CPR training and whenever possible, arrangements should be made to have a Board of Certification (BOC)-certified athletic trainer or other appropriate emergency care providers present at practices and games.
- Inspect the gymnasium for irregularities on the floor, including water or other liquids, and adequate lighting and ventilation.
- Use mouth guards to reduce the chance of dental injuries and concussions.
- Do not apply athletic tape to ankles or other joints without being trained in their correct application. If possible, seek the services of a BOC-certified athletic trainer.
- Athletes with a history of ankle problems should purchase a commercially manufactured ankle brace that fits correctly.
- Inspect shoes frequently to ensure good arch support and traction.
- Include 10 to 15 minutes of warm-up activity prior to play, including stretching the shoulder muscles, hamstrings, and Achilles tendon.
- Coaches and parents should stress properly supervised physical conditioning on a year-round basis, including during the season. Muscle strength in the extremities and trunk

is important to prevent strains and to protect joints from sprains. In addition, athletes should be instructed on proper stretching methods and focus on the Achilles tendons, hamstrings, and the muscles of the low back and shoulder regions.

- Athletes should be required to remove any jewelry such as rings, earrings, bracelets, and necklaces during both games and practices.

Football

Football, also called *tackle football* or *American football*, involves numerous collisions among players from opposing teams and often incidental contact among players from the same team during tackles. Although considerable protective equipment is required for personal safety, injuries are an accepted part of the game.

Most Common Football Injuries

- General trauma (bruises, abrasions)
- Sprains (joint injuries)
- Strains (muscle and tendon injuries)
- Concussions
- Fractures

Body Areas Injured in Football

- Ankle and foot
- Hip, thigh, and leg
- Shoulder, arm, and hand
- Knee
- Head, neck, and spine

Injury Prevention Guidelines for Football

- Coaches should be required to have current first aid and CPR training. Whenever possible, arrangements should be made to have a BOC-certified athletic trainer or other appropriate emergency care providers present at practices and games.
- Coaches and parents should require participants to perform properly supervised preseason conditioning exercises for muscle strength and flexibility of the shoulders, upper arms, and neck, and the trunk, hips and thighs, and ankles. Conditioning programs should be continued, albeit at a reduced level, throughout the playing season as well.

- Regularly inspect helmets, new and reconditioned, to ensure they are stamped with the National Operating Committee on Standards for Athletic Equipment (NOCSAE) seal.
- Helmets, chin straps, and shoulder pads must be sized correctly and adjusted for a good fit **Figure 6-2**.
- Use mouth guards to reduce the chance of dental injuries and concussions.
- Spearing should not be coached or allowed, because it can lead to catastrophic head and neck injuries.
- Teach athletes to block and tackle in the "head-up" position.
- Include 10 to 15 minutes of warm-up activities before play, including stretching the

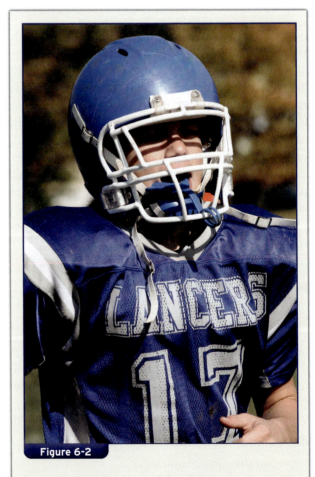

Figure 6-2

Be sure athletes' helmets fit correctly.

shoulders, low back, hips, thighs, and Achilles tendon muscles.
- Inspect the playing field for debris, irregularities, and length of grass.
- Do not apply athletic tape to the ankles or other joints of the body without having been trained in their correct application. If possible, seek the services of a BOC-certified athletic trainer.
- Athletes with a history of ankle problems should purchase a commercially manufactured ankle brace.

Ice Hockey

Ice hockey is a popular sport worldwide with a wide variance in rules governing the amount of contact allowed among players. A unique aspect of the game involves a maneuver known as *body checking*, in which a player intentionally collides with an opponent with the puck, using the hip or shoulder to force the player into the boards or to the ice. The American Academy of Pediatrics advises that body checking not be allowed for players 15 years old and younger to reduce the risk of serious injuries related to these collisions. In addition, the National Collegiate Athletic Association (NCAA) requires collegiate players to wear full-face protection and USA Hockey requires that junior players wear full-face protection.

Most Common Ice Hockey Injuries

- Contusions (bruises)
- Concussions
- Sprains (joint injuries)
- Strains (muscle and tendon injuries)
- Fractures and dislocations
- Wounds (lacerations and abrasions)

Body Areas Injured in Ice Hockey

- Head and face
- Upper extremities (shoulder, arm, hand, and wrist)
- Lower extremities (hip, thigh, knee, and ankle)

Injury Prevention Guidelines for Ice Hockey

- Coaches should be required to have current first aid and CPR training. Whenever possible, arrangements should be made to have a BOC-certified athletic trainer or other appropriate emergency care providers present at practices and games.
- Encourage properly supervised preseason conditioning exercises for the shoulders, upper arms, and neck, and the trunk, hips and thighs, and ankle strength and flexibility. Conditioning programs should be continued, albeit at a reduced level, throughout the playing season as well.
- Regularly inspect helmets, chin straps, faceguards, and throat protectors for proper fit, wear, and protection. Ensure that helmets meet the Hockey Equipment Certification Council (HECC) certification standards.
- Ensure that players wear all required protective equipment during practice and games. Players should be required, or strongly encouraged, to wear either partial or full face shields during games and practice regardless of age or skill level.
- Regularly inspect the ice for hazards such as deep ruts and gouges. Whenever possible, resurface the playing area.
- Use mouth guards to reduce the chance of dental injuries and concussions **Figure 6-3**.
- Ensure that all essential lines, such as the centerline, can be seen clearly below the surface of the ice.

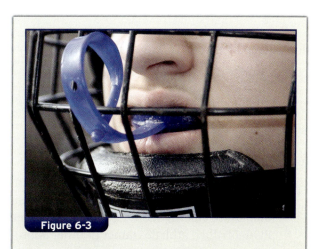

Figure 6-3

Mouth guards help protect against dental injuries and concussion.

- Perform 10 to 15 minutes of warm-up activities before play, stretching the muscles of the shoulders, lower back, hips, thighs, and Achilles tendon.
- Ensure that all rules pertaining to body and stick checking are strictly enforced during both practice and games.
- Make certain goals are not anchored.
- Encourage and reinforce "heads-up hockey" programs to prevent catastrophic head and neck injuries.

Lacrosse

As the oldest American sport, originally played by Native Americans, lacrosse continues to be very popular, especially at the community and college level. Although both genders can enjoy the game, the rules are different in that more physical contact between players is allowed in the men's game while women are not allowed to have body or stick contact with opponents. As such, protective equipment for men includes helmets; however, with the exception of the goalie, women are not required to wear helmets.

Most Common Lacrosse Injuries

- Fractures
- Strains (muscle and tendon injuries)
- Sprains (joint injuries)
- Contusions (bruises)
- Lacerations
- Concussions

Body Areas Injured in Lacrosse

- Finger
- Shoulder
- Elbow
- Ankle
- Knee

Injury Prevention Guidelines for Lacrosse

- Coaches should be required to have current first aid and CPR training. Whenever possible, arrangements should be made to have a BOC-certified athletic trainer or other appropriate emergency care providers present at practices and games.

- Inspect the playing field for debris, irregularities in the playing surface, and length of grass.
- Regularly inspect helmets, chin straps, and facemasks to ensure they are in good condition.
- All helmets, including women's goalie helmets, regardless of age category, should be certified as meeting the NOCSAE standards.
- As of January 1, 2005, the US Lacrosse Women's Division Board of Governors mandated that protective eye wear meet the ASTM F803-03, which states that protective eyewear should withstand forces generated by a ball traveling 45 miles per hour for youth play and 60 miles per hour for adult play (high school and older). A listing of products meeting this standard is available at the US Lacrosse web site.
- Encourage properly supervised preseason conditioning exercises for the shoulders, upper arms, and neck, and the trunk, hips and thighs, and ankle strength and flexibility. Conditioning programs should be continued, albeit at a reduced level, throughout the playing season as well.
- Helmets, arm and shoulder pads, and gloves must be sized correctly and properly adjusted for fit.
- Verify that goals, nets, and stands are constructed correctly and painted orange.
- Use mouth guards to reduce the chance of dental injuries and concussions.
- Perform 10 to 15 minutes of warm-up activities before play including stretching, jogging, swinging the stick, and catching the ball with the stick.
- Wear a sunscreen product on all body areas that are exposed to the sun, with special attention to the nose, lips, ears, base of the neck, and legs.
- Discontinue practice or a game in the event of threatening weather, such as a lightning storm or excessively high temperatures or humidity.
- Do not apply athletic tape to the ankles or other joints of the body without having been

trained in their correct application. If possible, seek the services of a BOC-certified athletic trainer.

- Athletes with a history of ankle problems should purchase a commercially manufactured ankle brace.
- Ensure that participants follow all rules regarding proper stick/body checking.

Martial Arts

Three martial arts sports in particular—judo, karate, and tae kwon do—have enjoyed tremendous growth over the past several decades in the United States. In both karate and tae kwon do, participants may contact their opponent with blows from either the feet or the hands. Judo utilizes various holds and throwing techniques and does not incorporate kicks and punches seen in other forms of martial arts. However, in spite of these differences, injuries do occur in judo, as well as the other forms, as a result of collisions and direct blows.

Most Common Martial Arts Injuries (by sport)

Judo
- Sprains (joint injuries)
- Bruises
- Strains

Karate and Tae Kwon Do
- Bruises (noncontact)
- Bruises (contact)
- Fractures
- Dental injuries
- Concussions

Body Areas Injured in Martial Arts

Judo
- Upper extremities
- Lower extremities
- Head, spine, and trunk

Karate
- Head, spine, and trunk
- Face

Tae Kwon Do
- Head, spine, and trunk
- Lower extremities

Injury Prevention Guidelines for Martial Arts

- Do not permit actual blows to an opponent at the beginner level in either karate or tae kwon do.
- Wear properly fitted clothing as per the requirements for that particular sport and keep the clothing clear and free of blood and other body fluids.
- Practice on safety mats that are designed for such use (judo).
- Clean practice areas regularly, including the mats, with a commercial solution to eliminate any microbes that may be present, avoiding transfer of skin infections among participants.
- Use closed fists and wear protective padding as required.
- Perform 10 to 15 minutes of warm-up activities prior to participation, including stretching the shoulder, spine, hip, thigh, Achilles tendon, ankle, and toe muscles.
- Have trained medical personnel such as a doctor, BOC-certified athletic trainer, or nurse available at all competitive venues. Instructors and coaches should be trained in first aid and CPR as well and when possible, these personnel should participate in additional training on topics focused on reducing injuries and improving the safety of participants.
- Consider rule modification to eliminate blows to the face and head in karate and tae kwon do.
- Use mouth guards to reduce the chance of dental injuries and concussions.

Roller Hockey

Roller hockey, also known as *inline hockey,* continues to grow in popularity in the United States as well as throughout the world. Roller hockey is similar to ice hockey, but does not allow checking, nor does it include off-sides play stoppages. Various skate types and designs can be utilized to include those known as *quads,* as well as inline. The game can be played with a puck or a ball. The risk of skate-related injuries is lower in roller hockey compared to ice hockey because in ice hockey the skate blades may come into contact with a participant, resulting in a laceration.

Most Common Roller Hockey Injuries

- Wounds (lacerations)
- Fractures
- Strains (muscle and tendon injuries)
- Sprains (joint injuries)
- Contusions (bruises)

Body Areas Injured in Roller Hockey

- Face
- Shoulder
- Knee
- Finger
- Lower leg
- Wrist

Injury Prevention Guidelines for Roller Hockey

- Coaches should be required to have current first aid and CPR training. Whenever possible, arrangements should be made to have a BOC-certified athletic trainer or other appropriate emergency care providers present at practices and games.
- Perform preseason conditioning exercises for shoulders, upper arms, and neck, and the trunk, hip and thigh, and ankle muscle strength and flexibility. Conditioning programs should be continued, albeit at a reduced level, throughout the playing season as well.
- Regularly inspect helmets, chin straps, and other safety equipment. Ensure that helmets have met the HECC certification standards.
- Given the number of facial injuries, face masks/guards are required.
- Ensure players are wearing all required protective equipment during both practice and games.
- Inspect the playing surface for ruts, holes, water, and cracks. Move to another venue when such conditions exist.
- Perform 10 to 15 minutes of warm-up activities prior to play, including stretching the

shoulder, lower back, hip, thigh, and Achilles tendon muscles.
- Rules regarding body checking, high sticking, and so forth must be strictly enforced.
- Be sure that the stick and blade conform to safety specifications.

Soccer

Soccer, the most popular sport worldwide, continues to attract millions of participants in organized play within the United States, with players ranging in age from the youth levels through adult, professional leagues. Many injuries are associated with hazardous playing field conditions, heading of the ball with poor technique, and techniques such as tackling from behind. Injuries to the ACL in female players increase significantly at age 14 years, and as such, preventative conditioning programs are critical at this age level. Although most soccer injuries involve the extremities and are minor in severity, some, such as head injuries related to collisions between players, can be serious. Another source of serious injuries and even death is the soccer goals. These injuries result from players colliding with unpadded goal posts or from unanchored goals tipping over and landing on a player.

Most Common Soccer Injuries

- General trauma (bruises and abrasions)
- Sprains (joint injuries)
- Strains (muscle and tendon injuries)

Body Areas Injured in Soccer

- Ankle and foot
- Hip, thigh, and leg
- Knee
- Torso
- Forearm, wrist, and hand

Injury Prevention Guidelines for Soccer

- Coaches should be required to have current first aid and CPR training. Whenever possible, arrangements should be made to have a BOC-certified athletic trainer or other appropriate emergency care providers present at practices and games.
- Encourage properly supervised preseason conditioning exercises for shoulders, upper

arms, and neck, and the trunk, hips and thighs, and ankle strength and flexibility. Conditioning programs should be continued, albeit at a reduced level, throughout the playing season as well.

- Inspect the playing field for debris, irregularities in the playing surface, and length of grass.
- Verify that goal posts, nets, and stands are secured correctly and meet league safety guidelines. It is highly recommended that goal posts be padded with a material that will decrease the impact forces associated with players colliding with the posts.
- Athletes should wear shin guards and proper shoes with correct cleats.
- Athletes should use mouth guards to reduce the chance of dental injuries and concussions.
- Perform 10 to 15 minutes of warm-up activities before play, including stretching, jogging, and kicking.
- Educate athletes regarding rules that apply to correct tackling techniques. Discourage slide tackles from behind an opponent.
- Athletes should wear a sunscreen on all body areas that are exposed to the sun, with special attention to the nose, lips, ears, base of neck, and arms **Figure 6-4** .
- Discontinue the practice or a game in the event of threatening weather, such as a lightning storm or excessively high temperatures or humidity.
- Any athlete who sustains an open wound must stop participating immediately. The wound must be cleaned and covered with a protective dressing. Bleeding must be controlled before the athlete returns to participation. Bloody uniforms must be changed prior to return to participation.

Wrestling

Wrestling has a huge following internationally, with over 2,900 wrestling clubs in the United States alone. Children as young as age 7 can compete in USA Wrestling–sanctioned events, with weight categories beginning at 40 lb. There are three primary styles of wrestling practiced by amateurs: freestyle,

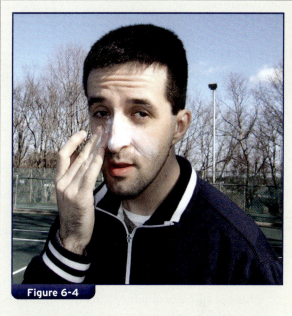

Figure 6-4

Athletes should apply sunscreen to any areas exposed to the sun.

Greco-Roman, and folkstyle which is the style incorporated at the interscholastic and intercollegiate levels in the United States. Wrestling enjoys considerable support due to the fact that it matches competitors on the basis of body weight so that smaller athletes are not forced to compete against those who have a significant size advantage.

Most Common Wrestling Injuries

- General trauma (bruises and abrasions)
- Strains (joint injuries)
- Sprains (muscle and tendon injuries)
- Skin disorders (infections from fungi, bacteria, and viruses)

Most Common Skin Conditions in Wrestling

- Ringworm (fungi)
- Impetigo (bacteria)
- Dermatitis
- Skin infection (bacteria)
- Herpes zoster (virus)

Body Areas Injured in Wrestling

- Forearm, wrist, and hand
- Shoulder and arm
- Knee

- Torso
- Head, neck, and spine

Injury Prevention Guidelines for Wrestling

- Coaches should be required to have current first aid and CPR training. Whenever possible, arrangements should be made to have a BOC-certified athletic trainer or other appropriate emergency care providers present at practices and competitions.
- Parents and athletes should be educated regarding weight loss in wrestling. To obtain the revised position paper *Weight Loss in Wrestlers* from the American College of Sports Medicine, send a stamped, self-addressed envelope to the following address: ACSM, P.O. Box 1440, Indianapolis, IN 46206-1440 (request this specific document). This document also is available online.
- Clean practice and competition mats frequently with an antiseptic solution (¼ cup bleach per gallon of water). If blood is on the mat, wrestling should be stopped immediately.
- When blood soaks into clothing, wrestling should be discontinued immediately and the clothing should be changed. Any blood on the skin should be removed with an antiseptic wipe before participation is allowed to resume. All bloody clothing, blood-soaked first aid materials, and the like should be handled according to bloodborne pathogen guidelines.
- According to USA Wrestling guidelines, no athletes known to be HIV positive can participate in a sanctioned event.
- Athletes should wear protective headgear, athletic supporter and cup (males), and knee pads **Figure 6-5**.
- Use mouth guards to reduce the chance of dental injuries and concussions.
- Practice good personal hygiene, including showering before and after practice.
- Regularly clean all protective equipment and clothing.
- Strongly discourage athletes from practicing rapid weight loss regimes.

- Ensure that athletes perform 10 to 15 minutes of warm-up activities before participating (stretching, jogging, etc.).

▶ Limited Contact Sports

Baseball/Softball

Baseball and softball continue to be extremely popular sports in the United States for both genders beginning with children as young as age 5. Overall, the majority of these children participate in both low and highly organized levels of play without sustaining serious injuries. However, a relatively low percentage of participants do suffer some level of injury each year. The majority of these injuries are contusions and abrasions that can be treated with simple first aid. However, more serious injuries can occur and are most often the outcome of a participant being struck by a batted ball, pitched ball, or bat. A severe blow to the chest region can result in cardiac arrest, known as *commotio cordis,* and has resulted in baseball- and softball-related deaths. In addition, severe head injuries can result when a base runner attempts a head-first sliding technique, resulting in a blow to the head. Eye injuries related to ball impacts also occur and the best protection is

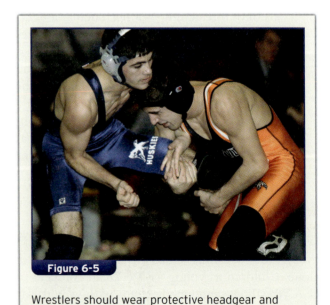

Figure 6-5

Wrestlers should wear protective headgear and knee pads.

to require that participants wear appropriate batting helmets with eye protection built in (see the following injury prevention guidelines).

Most Common Baseball/Softball Injuries

- General trauma (bruises and abrasions)
- Strains (muscle and tendon injuries)
- Sprains (joint injuries)

Body Areas Injured in Baseball/Softball

- Forearm, wrist, and hand
- Shoulder and arm
- Hip, thigh, and leg
- Face and scalp (including the eyes)
- Ankle and foot

Injury Prevention Guidelines for Baseball/Softball

- Coaches should be required to have current first aid and CPR training and whenever possible, arrangements should be made to have a BOC-certified athletic trainer or other appropriate emergency care providers present at practices and competitions.
- Proper conditioning is essential and should include strength and flexibility exercises for the shoulder, trunk, and legs. In addition, participants should receive proper instruction on throwing technique.
- The conditioning program should include the muscles of the back of the shoulder responsible for slowing the arm after throwing (rotator cuff).
- Rules should limit the number of innings pitched per consecutive calendar days.
- As recommended by the American Academy of Pediatrics, age-appropriate balls should be used (eg, low-impact NOCSAE-approved baseballs/softballs for children 5 to 14 years old).
- Rules regarding head-first sliding into bases should be strictly enforced.
- Stronger, physically mature athletes should exercise caution when throwing or batting to younger, less-physically mature players. There are numerous accounts of deaths in younger players resulting from being struck in the chest or head by a thrown or batted

ball. Catchers should be required to wear all necessary protective equipment, including a chest protector.
- Gradually warm up the major muscle groups of the body, including the shoulder, low back, hamstrings, and Achilles tendon.
- Batters must wear required protective equipment, including a batting helmet with polycarbonate face shield.
- Inspect safety fencing behind home plate, the playing field surface, bases, and the location of players' benches or dugouts relative to the batting area.
- Inspect the playing field for debris, irregularities, and length of grass.
- Inspect equipment such as helmets and bats before use in practice or games. Damaged equipment should be discarded and replaced.
- Wear a sunscreen product on all body areas that are exposed to the sun, with special attention to the nose, lips, ears, neck, and arms.
- Discontinue practice or game during threatening weather such as a lightning storm or excessively high or low temperatures.
- Do not wear jewelry such as rings, earrings, bracelets, or necklaces, because they may cause crush or amputation injuries.
- Wear appropriate footwear that is safe for the level of play.
- Use break-away bases.

> **CAUTION**
>
> Baseball and softball players should be careful when throwing or batting to players who are not as physically strong. The resulting hit could cause severe injury.

Cheerleading

Since the early 1980s, college- and high school–level cheerleading has evolved from game-related entertainment designed to elevate team spirit and fan support into its own competitive sport. To be competitive, cheerleaders must possess and refine numerous athletic abilities and skills similar to those of competitive gymnasts and dancers. As cheerleading has become more competitive, the number and severity of injuries has increased dramatically. Although both genders participate in cheerleading, the vast majority of those injured are female. Deaths and permanent injury, most often related to head and/or neck injury, have been reported and historically been related to highly dangerous activities such as jumping off mini-trampolines, or when performing pyramid formations where participants accidentally fall or are dropped.

Most Common Cheerleading Injuries

- Strains (muscle and tendon injuries)
- Sprains (joint injuries)
- Lacerations
- Contusions (bruises)
- Dislocations

Body Areas Injured in Cheerleading

- Ankle
- Lower trunk
- Wrist, hand, and fingers
- Knee
- Face
- Head and neck

Injury Prevention Guidelines for Cheerleading

- A qualified coach with training in gymnastics and expertise in correct spotting techniques should train cheerleaders. Coaching personnel should be required to have a valid first aid and CPR card.
- Cheerleading coaches should have some type of safety certification, such as that offered by the American Association of Cheerleading Coaches and Administrators.
- Cheerleaders should undergo proper conditioning programs that include proper spotting technique components.
- Only cheerleaders with proper training should attempt gymnastic-type stunts. A qualification system demonstrating mastery of stunts is recommended.
- Coaches should supervise all practice sessions in a safe facility **Figure 6-6**.

- Mini-trampolines and flips or falls off pyramids and shoulders should be prohibited.
- Pyramids over two persons high should not be performed. Two-person-high pyramids should be performed only with mats and spotters.
- If it is not possible to have a doctor or BOC-certified athletic trainer at games and practice sessions, emergency procedures must be provided and available in writing to staff and athletes.
- When a cheerleader has experienced or shows signs of head or neck trauma (loss of consciousness, visual disturbances, headache, inability to walk correctly, obvious disorientation, memory loss, or numbness in one or more of the extremities), he or she should receive immediate medical care and should not be allowed back to practice without permission from appropriate medical authorities.

Field Events

Track and field throwing and jumping events (known as *field events*) continue to attract participants within the United States, particularly at the high school and college levels. Severe and catastrophic injuries are rare. When they do occur, they usually are related to landing incorrectly in the pole vault pit, or to javelin

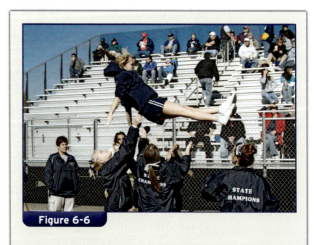

Figure 6-6

Coaches should supervise all practice sessions in a safe facility.

and discus events. Spectators can be injured by a javelin, shot put, hammer, or discus when throwing areas are not adequately managed to avoid situations in which spectators can access the landing areas for these objects. In addition, it is critical that athletes be constantly reminded to exercise extreme care during practices to avoid walking into a landing area when other athletes are throwing. Most of these injuries are preventable through close event supervision and careful attention to the placement of safety fences or lines for both spectators and participants.

Most Common Field Events Injuries

- Strains (muscle and tendon injuries)
- Sprains (joint injuries)
- Stress fractures
- Nerve injuries
- Injuries to immature bone (major tendon attachments)

Body Areas Injured in Field Events

- Head, spine, and trunk
- Shoulder
- Elbow
- Knee
- Ankle and foot

Injury Prevention Guidelines for Field Events

- Coaches should be required to have current first aid and CPR training. Whenever possible, arrangements should be made to have a BOC-certified athletic trainer or other appropriate emergency care providers present at practices and competitions.
- Perform preseason conditioning exercises for muscle strength and flexibility of the shoulders, upper arms, and neck, and the trunk, hips and thighs, and ankles. Give special attention to the muscle in the back of the shoulder (rotator cuff) in throwers, and the knee and lower leg muscles in jumpers.
- In throwing events, make sure all spectators and nonparticipants stay within well-marked safety lines or retaining fences.
- Consider using safer implements, such as rubber-tipped javelins and rubber discus, during practice.

- Include 10 to 15 minutes of warm-up activities prior to participation, stretching the shoulder muscles, lower back, hips and thighs, Achilles tendon, and ankles.
- In jumping events, especially the high jump and pole vault, the landing pits should be designed and maintained to ensure safe landings. All framing material should be covered with high-density foam rubber to prevent injury if an athlete lands on the pit's edge.
- Pole vaulters should use poles rated at their body weight.
- Wear a sunscreen product on all exposed body areas, paying special attention to the nose, lips, ears, neck, arms, and legs.
- Wear the correct footwear for the event.

Gymnastics

In the United States, a fairly small number of males participate in gymnastics while the vast majority of participants are females. Presently, the majority of youth participants are at the club level with a far smaller number of athletes associated with competitive programs at the collegiate level. Gymnastics is a sport that puts a premium on very young participants, with elite-level participants typically ranging in age from 12 to 18 years old. USA Gymnastics, the national governing body for gymnastics in the United States, has developed an extensive program of coaching certification and safety training.

Most Common Gymnastics Injuries

- Sprains (joint injuries)
- Strains (muscle and tendon injuries)
- General trauma (bruises and abrasions)
- Fractures

Body Areas Injured in Gymnastics

- Ankle
- Elbow
- Finger
- Wrist
- Lower arm (forearm)
- Spine (particularly the low back) and trunk

Injury Prevention Guidelines for Gymnastics

- Coaches should be required to have current first aid and CPR training. Whenever possible, arrangements should be made to have a BOC-certified athletic trainer or other appropriate emergency care providers present at practices and competitions.
- Perform 10 to 15 minutes of warm-up activities before participating, including stretching the shoulders, low back, hips, thighs, Achilles tendon, and ankle muscles.
- Athletes should always practice with a spotter, preferably a qualified coach.
- Avoid successive practice sessions that include repeated cycles of dismounts.
- Follow heavy workouts with a day or more of reduced intensity training.
- Regularly inspect all apparatus and safety equipment including mats, crash pads, spotting belts and associated ropes, pulleys, and so forth.
- Athletes should report persistent pain in any body region, especially in the lower back, hips, and knees.

Skiing (Alpine)

Alpine (downhill) skiing continues to enjoy widespread participation within the United States. The vast majority of participants are at the recreational level with a smaller number involved in competitive ski racing beginning at the youth level. Although overall alpine skiing is a relatively safe sport, injuries do occur. The majority of injuries are related to falls resulting in injuries to the extremities. Head and neck injuries can occur, sometimes related to collisions with other skiers or impacts with obstacles such as trees or rocks.

Most Common Alpine Skiing Injuries

- Sprains (joint injuries)
- Fractures
- Dislocations
- Strains (muscle and tendon injuries)

Body Areas Injured in Skiing

- Knee
- Shoulder
- Thumb
- Head and spine

Injury Prevention Guidelines for Alpine Skiing

- Athletes should receive instruction from a certified ski instructor at the beginning of each ski season.
- Ski instruction should include avoiding behaviors that place the knee at a high risk of injury.
- Ensure that all ski equipment is inspected by a certified ski mechanic at the beginning of each season.
- Initiate a preseason conditioning program that focuses on muscle strength in the legs, trunk, and shoulders.
- Ski with equipment at the appropriate ability level. Wear a helmet designed for alpine skiing. In addition, properly fitted goggles designed for alpine sports also should be worn.
- Test bindings' release mechanisms at the beginning of each ski day.
- Teach athletes to ski with control and to stop skiing when tired.
- Be familiar with the ski area and the difficulty level of the runs.

Volleyball

Variations of volleyball are popular worldwide with the most well-known form of the game, commonly referred to as *power volleyball,* played in the public schools and colleges in the United States. There are popular variations of the sport, such as beach volleyball, which is played on a sand surface rather than the more traditional indoor playing surface, typically a hardwood floor.

Most Common Volleyball Injuries

- Sprains (joint injuries)
- Strains (muscle and tendon injuries)
- General trauma (bruises and abrasions)
- Fractures

Body Areas Injured in Volleyball

- Ankle and foot
- Hip, thigh, and leg
- Forearm, wrist, and hand

- Knee
- Shoulder and arm

Injury Prevention Guidelines for Volleyball

- Coaches should be required to have current first aid and CPR training. Whenever possible, arrangements should be made to have a BOC-certified athletic trainer or other appropriate emergency care providers present at practices and games.
- Inspect the gymnasium with respect to irregularities on the floor including water or other fluids, lighting, and ventilation.
- Ensure that the net support structures and referee stand are well padded to protect players.
- Avoid play on concrete or synthetic floor surfaces.
- Athletes should be coached on proper jumping and landing techniques.
- Proper conditioning is essential and should include exercises to increase strength and flexibility in the muscles of the shoulders, hips, knees, and ankles.
- Do not apply athletic tape to the ankles or other joints of the body without proper training in their correct application. If possible, seek the services of a BOC-certified athletic trainer.
- Athletes with a history of ankle problems should purchase a commercially manufactured ankle brace.
- Wear protective kneepads during both practice and games.
- Educate athletes regarding the dangers of collisions with teammates.
- Inspect shoes frequently to ensure ankle support and shock absorption.
- Include 10 to 15 minutes of warm-up activities before play, including stretching the muscles of the shoulder, hamstrings, and Achilles tendon.

▶ Noncontact Sports

Swimming

Competitive swimming is immensely popular in the United States, with millions of participants of all ages.

Competitive swimming programs are offered through a variety of venues, including public schools, YMCAs and YWCAs, and extensive community-based programs and clubs. In general, participant safety is a major priority associated with aquatic programs. As such, there are fairly few traumatic injuries associated with competitive swimming programs. Virtually all public pools benefit from having trained lifeguards on duty during both recreational and competitive swimming events.

By far, the majority of swimming injuries are related to overtraining. These are typically called *overuse injuries*. Most of these injuries occur from an incorrect stroke technique, excessive training, or injuries aggravated by other types of training such as weight training.

Most Common Swimming Injuries

- Strains (muscle and tendon injuries)
- Sprains (joint injuries)
- Infections (bacterial, viral, and fungal)

Body Areas Injured in Swimming

- Shoulder
- Elbow
- Ankle
- Back
- Ear (internal infections)

Injury Prevention Guidelines for Swimming

- Coaches should be required to have current first aid and CPR training. Whenever possible, arrangements should be made to have a BOC-certified athletic trainer or other appropriate emergency care providers present at practices and competitions.
- Stress safety to all participants whenever in or around the pool.
- Athletes should be coached to perform swimming strokes correctly.
- While warming up and stretching are important, caution should be exercised to avoid excessive and potentially injurious stretching, especially partner stretching.
- Avoid overtraining. A typical sign of overtraining is a sudden, unexplained decline in swimming performance.

- Training programs should be structured to incorporate sufficient rest to allow adequate recovery between difficult training sessions.
- Wear a swim cap to avoid ear infections **Figure 6-7** .
- After swimming, treat ears with a few drops of solution, such as isopropranol (isopropyl alcohol). Alcohol is heavier than water and dries out the ear canal, thus preventing ear infections.
- Do not swim when an active skin infection is present.
- To avoid eye irritation, wear properly fitted goggles.
- Maintain lines of communication among the coach, athlete, and parents.
- In competitive swimming, strictly enforce the proper use of starting blocks.
- Make sure swimmers understand circle swimming procedures during practice.
- Do not allow any horseplay around the deck. Swimmers often are injured running on wet, slick surfaces, and by throwing kickboards.

Tennis

Tennis is a very popular racquet sport in the United States and Europe. Tennis is played in the community and in private clubs, public schools, colleges, and at the professional level.

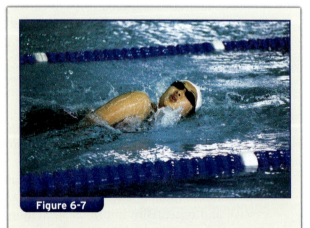

Figure 6-7

Use of a swim cap and goggles reduces the risk of ear infections and eye irritation.

Most Common Tennis Injuries

- Sprains (joint injuries)
- Strains (muscle and tendon injuries)
- Heat-related injuries (cramps, heat exhaustion, and heat stroke)

Body Areas Injured in Tennis

- Trunk
- Upper extremities (shoulder and elbow)
- Lower extremities (knee, lower leg, and Achilles tendon)

Injury Prevention Guidelines for Tennis

- Coaches should be required to have current first aid and CPR training. Whenever possible, arrangements should be made to have a BOC-certified athletic trainer or other appropriate emergency care providers present at practices and matches.
- Perform a preseason conditioning program for general muscle strength throughout the body, emphasizing the back of the shoulder muscles. Include 10 to 15 minutes of warm-up activities prior to play, stretching the muscles of the shoulders, lower back, hips, thighs, and Achilles tendon.
- Extend the warm-up period to include on-court warm-ups by hitting the ball lightly to an opponent in all major strokes: overhead, forehand, and backhand.
- Do not apply athletic tape to the ankles or other joints of the body without having been trained in their correct application.
- Athletes with a history of ankle problems should purchase a commercially manufactured ankle brace. If possible, seek the services of a BOC-certified athletic trainer.
- Inspect shoes frequently to ensure adequate foot support and shock absorption.
- Teach athletes to avoid gripping the racquet too tightly, especially for prolonged periods.
- Athletes should seek medical care for persistent pain in high-risk areas such as the elbow, shoulder, or lower back.
- Athletes should wear sunscreen on all body areas that are exposed to the sun, with spe-

cial attention to the nose, lips, ears, base of neck, arms, and legs.

- Parents and coaches should avoid placing undue pressure on young athletes.

Track

Running events in track and field include sprints, middle-distance, and distance events, as well as hurdles events. Running events are safe overall and result in few injuries; when injuries do occur, they typically involve the lower extremities or are related to falls in events such as the hurdles.

Most Common Track Injuries

- Strains (muscle and tendon injuries)
- Sprains (joint injuries)
- Shin splints (pain associated with the lower leg bones)

Body Areas Injured in Track

- Lower leg (shin)
- Ankle
- Knee
- Thigh
- Lower back

Injury Prevention Guidelines for Track

- Coaches should be required to have current first aid and CPR training. Whenever possible, arrangements should be made to have a BOC-certified athletic trainer or other appropriate emergency care providers present at practices and competitions.
- Perform preseason conditioning exercises for strength and flexibility in the muscles of the shoulder, upper arms, and neck, and the trunk, hips and thighs, and ankles. Special attention should be given to the muscles of the thigh (hamstrings and quadriceps), as well as the lower leg and ankle.
- Before any running events, perform 10 to 15 minutes of warm-up activities to stretch the muscles of the low back, hips, thighs (hamstrings), Achilles tendons, and ankles. Warm-ups should include jogging and brief sprints.
- Shin splints (persistent pain along the shin) or other leg pain that persists for more than

a few days should be evaluated by a BOC-certified athletic trainer or licensed doctor.

- Avoid overtraining. A typical sign of overtraining is a sudden, unexplained decline in running performance, which is especially important for middle-distance and distance runners.
- Training programs should be structured to incorporate sufficient rest to allow adequate recovery between difficult training sessions. Periods of recovery should be built into the overall training program for any track athlete.
- Wear sunscreen on all body areas that are exposed to the sun, with special attention to the nose, lips, ears, base of neck, arms, and legs.
- Wear the correct footwear for the event and the running surface.
- Hurdle practice should be conducted on areas of the track away from other participants to avoid collisions between runners and displaced hurdles **Figure 6-8**.

Weight Lifting and Weight Training

Weight lifting has evolved into a highly competitive sport, and depending on the specific types of lifts, is known as either power lifting (bench press, dead lift, squat) or Olympic lifting (snatch and the clean and jerk). Weight training involves the use of many

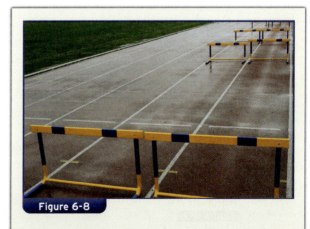

Figure 6-8

To avoid collision, hurdle practice should be conducted away from other runners.

types of lifts and available equipment to improve muscle strength, power, and/or physical appearance.

Most Common Weight-Lifting and Weight-Training Injuries

Weight Lifting
- Sprains (joint injuries)
- Strains (muscle and tendon injuries)
- Chronic injuries (strains, arthritis, etc.)

Weight Training
- Strains (muscle and tendon injuries)
- Sprains (joint injuries)
- Bruises
- Abrasions
- Fractures

Body Areas Injured in Weight Lifting and Weight Training

Weight Lifting
- Knees
- Shoulders
- Elbows
- Wrists
- Lower back

Weight Training
- Fingers
- Trunk
- Shoulders
- Face
- Toes

Injury Prevention Guidelines for Weight Lifting and Weight Training

- For proper recovery, avoid exercising the same muscle groups every day. The process of incorporating adequate recovery time in a training program is critical to allow the body time to respond to the training program by improving overall strength. As a general rule, a minimum of 24 hours should be allowed for recovery in any muscle group that has undergone intense strength training.
- For heavy lifting, consider using a weight belt **Figure 6-9** .
- Athletes should obtain proper instruction for performing each lift. This is especially critical for more complex free-weight lifts such as Olympic lifts. Injuries can occur when per-

forming free-weight exercises unless proper technique is used.
- Make sure weight collars are in place and functional when using free weight barbells. Athletes should lift only in designated areas of the facility that are designed for lifting to avoid collisions with other lifters.
- When using safety devices such as squat racks, make sure they are properly adjusted to the height of the lifter.
- When lifting moderate to heavy weights in exercises such as the bench press, make sure experienced spotters are always present.
- Proper warm-up is essential to avoid muscle/tendon injuries. Warm-ups should include stretching major muscle groups, as well as light, low-weight lifting prior to heavier lifts.
- Weight-training facilities should be designed to provide adequate space between all lifting stations.
- With younger lifters, avoid workouts that last longer than 30 to 45 minutes.
- Children and young adults should be educated as to the importance of avoiding ergogenic aids such as creatine, "andro," growth hormones, and anabolic steroids.
- Children and young adults should always be supervised when lifting.
- Do not allow adolescents and preadolescents to engage in 1 RPM lifts because these can re-

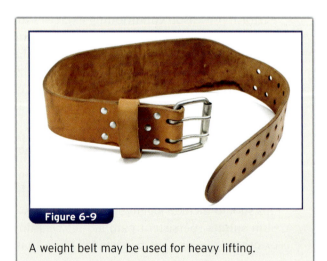

Figure 6-9

A weight belt may be used for heavy lifting.

sult in injury, particularly in young children. Avoid making weight training competitive in these age groups as well. As a general rule, all lifts should incorporate a protocol of moderation whereby the child never exceeds a weight that cannot be lifted 8–12 repetitions in each set of exercises. The National Strength and Conditioning Association (NSCA) has developed a position paper that addresses strength training in children; it can be obtained by visiting the NSCA web site.

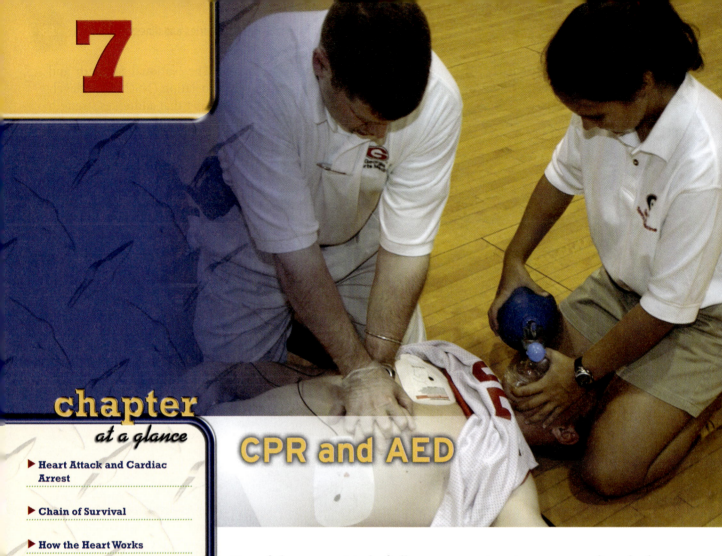

7

chapter
at a glance

▶ Heart Attack and Cardiac Arrest

▶ Chain of Survival

▶ How the Heart Works

▶ Care for Cardiac Arrest

▶ Performing CPR

▶ Airway Obstruction

▶ Public Access Defibrillation

▶ About AEDs

▶ Using an AED

▶ Special Considerations

▶ AED Maintenance

▶ Summary

CPR and AED

One of the most critical of all emergency situations occurs when the heart loses its ability to pump blood effectively. While this situation is more common in adults with underlying heart disease, it may also occur suddenly in athletes with undiagnosed heart disorders and those suffering from other acute conditions such as severe trauma, breathing disorders, and other medical emergencies. Rapid early intervention to restore blood flow to vital organs, such as the brain (chest compressions and artificial respirations), and methods to regain normal electrical activity in the heart (electrical defibrillation) can dramatically improve survival in many of these cases. This chapter focuses on heart conditions and cardiac arrest as they relate to the athlete and any person a coach may encounter (such as a referee, bystander, or other coach) during the course of a sporting event or at any time.

▶ Heart Attack and Cardiac Arrest

Although heart attacks are uncommon in young athletes, it is important for the youth coach to understand the signs and symptoms of a heart attack and the actions to take if someone experiences symptoms of a heart-related condition. Coaches should always consider the underlying causes if a heart-related condition affects a young athlete. Although it is not the role of the coach to determine the true cause of the health issue, the coach may be able to provide important information to medical personnel, which subsequently can affect the outcome of the event. A cardiac-related event must be considered in any victim, especially young athletes, who collapses suddenly without prior signs and symptoms.

A *heart attack* occurs when heart muscle tissue dies because its blood supply is severely reduced or stopped. This often occurs because of a clot in one or more coronary arteries. If damage to the heart muscle is too severe, the victim's heart can stop beating—a condition known as *cardiac arrest*. Sudden cardiac arrest is a leading cause of death in the United States, affecting about 250,000 people yearly in out-of-hospital locations. Common causes of cardiac events in younger individuals are listed in Table 7-1 .

▶ Chain of Survival

Few victims experiencing sudden cardiac arrest outside of a hospital survive unless a rapid sequence of events takes place. The chain of survival is a way of describing the ideal sequence of care that should take place when a cardiac arrest occurs Figure 7-1 .

The five links in the chain of survival are as follows:

1. **Early access:** Recognizing the emergency and immediately calling 9-1-1 or other local emergency number to activate EMS.

Table 7-1 Possible Causes of Heart Problems in Youth Athletes

Traumatic Causes	History	Presenting Signs and Symptoms	Treatment
Commotio Cordis	Blow to chest. Consider if athlete was struck in the chest with a baseball, hockey puck, lacrosse ball, or other object.	Sudden collapse within seconds or minutes after blow to the chest	Call 9-1-1. Follow CPR/AED protocols.
Cardiac Contusion	Any blow to the chest.	Chest pain Weakness and dizziness Feels like heart is skipping a beat	Call 9-1-1. Treat as if a heart attack.
Medical Causes	History	Presenting Signs and Symptoms	Treatment
Underlying heart condition	Usually none.	Sudden collapse	Call 9-1-1. Follow CPR/AED protocols.
Drug ingestion (question fellow athletes regarding the use of illicit or prescription drugs)	Recent ingestion of drug. Consider the use of amphetamines, cocaine, steroids, and other performance-enhancing substances.	Sudden collapse Chest pain Vomiting Palpitations Altered level of responsiveness Unusual or atypical behavior Dizziness Seizures	Call 9-1-1. Treat according to symptoms. If unconscious or unresponsive, use CPR/AED protocols.
Breathing problems (such as asthma)	Chest discomfort or pain.	Consider if preceded by shortness of breath	Treat according to symptoms.

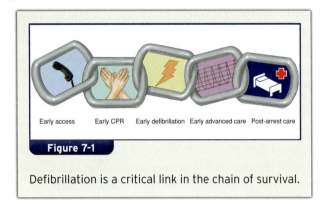

Figure 7-1

Defibrillation is a critical link in the chain of survival.

Early access   Early CPR   Early defibrillation   Early advanced care   Post-arrest care

2. **Early CPR:** Cardiopulmonary resuscitation supplies a minimal amount of blood to the heart and brain. It buys time until a defibrillator and EMS personnel are available. It can double or triple the victim's chances of survival.

3. **Early defibrillation:** Administering a shock to the heart using an automated external defibrillator (AED) can restore the heartbeat in some victims. It can produce survival rates as high as 50% to 75%.

4. **Early advanced care:** Health care providers give advanced cardiac life support to victims of sudden cardiac arrest. This includes providing IV fluids, medications, and advanced airway devices.

5. **Post-arrest care:** The hospital can provide lifesaving medications, surgical procedures, and advanced medical care to enable the victim of sudden cardiac arrest to survive and recover.

If any one of these links in the chain is broken (absent), the chance that the victim will survive is greatly decreased. If all links in the chain are strong, the victim has the best possible chance of survival.

TIP

Defibrillation
Most adults in cardiac arrest need defibrillation. Early defibrillation is the single most important factor in surviving cardiac arrest.

▶ How the Heart Works

The *heart* is an organ with four hollow chambers. The two chambers on the right side receive blood from the body and send it to the lungs for oxygen. The two chambers on the left side of the heart receive freshly oxygenated blood from the lungs and send it out to the body.

The heart has a unique electrical system that controls the rate at which the heart beats, as well as the amount of work the heart performs. In the right upper chamber of the heart, there is a collection of special pacemaker cells. About 60 to 100 times a minute, these cells emit electrical impulses that cause the other heart muscle cells to contract in a coordinated manner **Figure 7-2**.

Because the heart contracts approximately every second, it needs an abundant supply of oxygen, which it gets through the coronary arteries. These arteries run along the outside of the heart muscle and branch into smaller vessels. These arteries sometimes become diseased (with atherosclerosis), resulting in a lack of oxygen to the pacemaker cells, which can cause abnormal electrical activity in the heart.

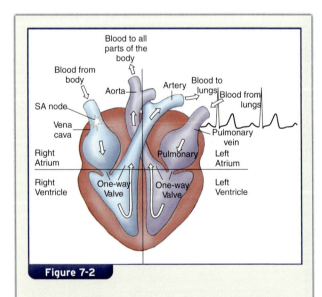

Figure 7-2

The sinoatrial (SA) node is the primary heart pacemaker, which sends electrical impulses to contract the heart's chambers in a coordinated manner.

When Normal Electrical Activity Is Interrupted

Ventricular fibrillation (also known as *V-fib*) is the most common abnormal heart rhythm in cases of sudden cardiac arrest in adults. The organized wave of electrical impulses that causes the heart muscle to contract and relax in a regular fashion is lost when the heart is in ventricular fibrillation. As a result, the lower chambers of the heart quiver and cannot pump blood, so circulation is lost (there is no pulse). A second, potentially life-threatening, electrical problem is *ventricular tachycardia* (*V-tach*), in which the heart beats too fast to pump blood effectively.

▶ Care for Cardiac Arrest

When the heart stops beating, the blood stops circulating, cutting off all oxygen and nourishment to the entire body. In this situation, time is a crucial factor. For every minute that defibrillation is delayed, the victim's chance of survival decreases by 7% to 10% **Figure 7-3**. CPR is the initial care for cardiac arrest until a defibrillator is available. Perform cycles of chest compressions and breaths until an AED is ready to be connected to the victim.

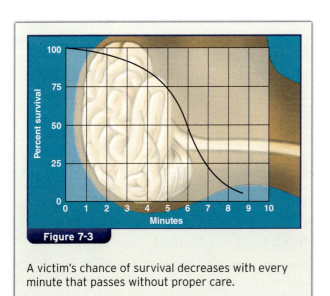

Figure 7-3

A victim's chance of survival decreases with every minute that passes without proper care.

▶ Performing CPR

When a person's heart stops beating, he or she needs CPR, an AED, and EMS professionals quickly. CPR consists of breathing oxygen into a victim's lungs and moving blood to the heart and brain by giving chest compressions. CPR techniques are very similar for children (ages 1–8) and adults (age 8 and older), with only a few slight variations based on the size of the victim.

Check for Responsiveness

In a motionless victim, check for responsiveness by tapping the victim's shoulder and asking if he or she is okay. If the victim does not respond, he or she is said to be unresponsive.

At the same time you check for responsiveness, you should look at the victim to see if he or she is breathing **Figure 7-4**. If the victim is not breathing or only gasping, EMS professionals are needed. Ask a bystander to call 9-1-1. If you are alone with an adult victim and a phone is nearby, call 9-1-1 yourself. If you are alone with a child or infant, give CPR for 2 minutes; then call 9-1-1.

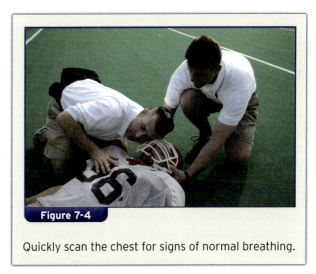

Figure 7-4

Quickly scan the chest for signs of normal breathing.

Give Chest Compressions

Chest compressions are the most important step in CPR. Perform chest compressions with two hands for an adult, one or two hands for a child, and two fingers for an infant. Effective compressions require rescuers to push hard and push fast. The chest of an adult should be compressed at least 2 inches; the chest of a child about 2 inches; and the chest of an infant about 1½ inches. The desired position for chest compressions is in the center of the chest.

Give compressions at a rate of at least 100 compressions per minute for adults, children, and infants. Give 30 compressions in about 18 seconds and then give two rescue breaths. Continue CPR until an AED becomes available, the victim shows signs of life, EMS personnel take over, or you are too tired to continue. Interruptions in compressions should be kept to a minimum.

Rescue Breaths

If the victim is not breathing, provide rescue breaths. With the airway open, pinch the victim's nose and using the mouth, make a tight seal over the victim's mouth. Give one breath lasting 1 second, take a normal breath (not a deep breath), and then give another breath like the first one. Each rescue breath should make the victim's chest rise. Other methods of rescue breathing are as follows:

- Mouth-to-barrier device
- Mouth-to-nose method
- Mouth-to-stoma method

Mouth-to-Barrier Device

A barrier device is placed in the victim's mouth or over the victim's mouth and nose as a precaution against infection. There are several different types

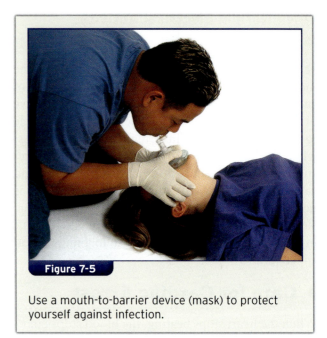

Figure 7-5

Use a mouth-to-barrier device (mask) to protect yourself against infection.

CAUTION

Coaches DO NOT:
- Check for a pulse or other signs of circulation (for example, movement) unless you are trained.
- Use a jaw thrust to open the airway unless you are trained in this method.

of barrier devices (for example, face shields and face masks), and all are easy to use with little modification to the mouth-to-mouth method **Figure 7-5**.

Mouth-to-Nose Method

If the victim's mouth cannot be opened, the jaw is clenched shut, the mouth is severely injured, or a good seal cannot be made with the victim's mouth, use the mouth-to-nose method. With the head tilted back, push up on the victim's chin to close the mouth. The rescuer should make a seal with their mouth over the victim's nose and provide rescue breaths.

Mouth-to-Stoma Method

Some diseases of the vocal cords result in surgical removal of the larynx. People who have this surgery breathe through a small, permanent opening in the

TIP

Avoiding Stomach Distention
Rescue breaths can cause stomach distention. Minimize this problem by limiting the breaths to the amount needed to make the chest rise. Avoid overinflating the victim's lungs by simply taking a normal breath yourself before breathing into the victim. Gastric distention can cause regurgitation of stomach contents and complicate care.

neck called a *stoma*. To perform mouth-to-stoma breathing, close the victim's mouth and nose and breathe through the opening in the neck.

Over the years, CPR procedures have changed, becoming easier for people to learn and remember. To perform adult CPR, follow the steps in **Skill Drill 7-1**:

1. Check responsiveness by tapping the victim and asking, "Are you okay?" If the victim is unresponsive, roll him or her onto his or her back. Quickly scan the victim's chest for signs of normal breathing (Step ❶).
2. Have someone call 9-1-1 or the local emergency number and retrieve an AED if available (Step ❷).
3. Begin CPR, starting with chest compressions.
   a. Place the heel of one hand on the center of the chest between the nipples. Place the other hand on top of the first hand (Step ❸).
   b. Depress the chest at least 2".
   c. Give 30 chest compressions at a rate of at least 100 per minute for an adult. Each set of 30 compressions should take about 18 seconds.
4. Open the airway using the head tilt–chin lift maneuver. Provide two rescue breaths of 1 second each, making the chest rise (Step ❹).
5. Continue cycles of 30 chest compressions and two ventilations until an AED becomes available, the victim is breathing, EMS takes over, or the rescuer is too exhausted to continue.

To perform CPR on a child, follow the steps in **Skill Drill 7-2**:

1. Check responsiveness by tapping the victim and asking, "Are you okay?" If the victim is unresponsive, roll him or her onto his or her back. Quickly scan the victim's chest for signs of normal breathing. Have someone call 9-1-1 or the local emergency number and retrieve an AED if available (Step ❶).

2. Begin CPR, starting with chest compressions.
   a. Place the heel of one hand on the center of the chest between the nipples. Place the other hand on top of the first hand (Step ❷).
   b. Depress the chest about 2".
   c. Give 30 chest compressions at a rate of at least 100 per minute. Each set of 30 compressions should take about 18 seconds.
3. Open the airway using the head tilt–chin lift maneuver.
4. Give two rescue breaths of 1 second each, making the chest rise (Step ❸).
5. Continue cycles of 30 chest compressions and two ventilations until an AED becomes available, the victim is breathing, EMS takes over, or the rescuer is too exhausted to continue.

skill drill

7-1   Adult CPR

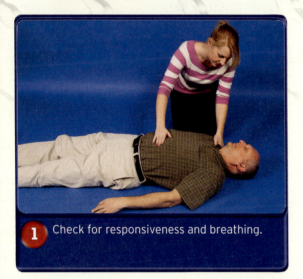

1 Check for responsiveness and breathing.

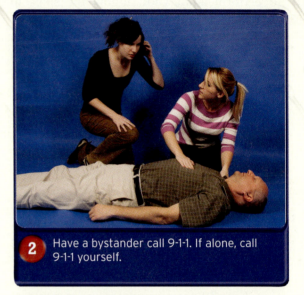

2 Have a bystander call 9-1-1. If alone, call 9-1-1 yourself.

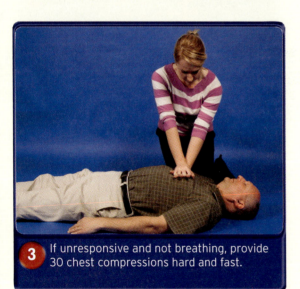

3 If unresponsive and not breathing, provide 30 chest compressions hard and fast.

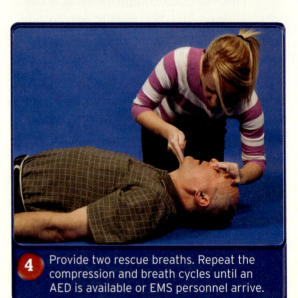

4 Provide two rescue breaths. Repeat the compression and breath cycles until an AED is available or EMS personnel arrive.

skill drill

7-2 Child CPR

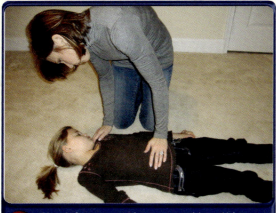

1 Check for responsiveness and breathing. Have a bystander call 9-1-1. If alone, call 9-1-1 yourself.

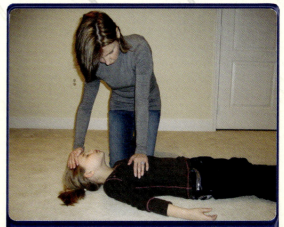

2 If the victim is unresponsive and not breathing, provide 30 chest compressions using one hand or two, depending on the size of the child.

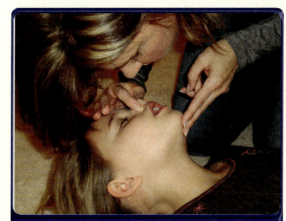

3 Provide two rescue breaths. Repeat the compression and breath cycles until an AED is available or EMS personnel arrive.

TIP

Compression-Only CPR

Mouth-to-mouth rescue breathing has a long safety record for victims and rescuers, but fear of infectious diseases causes some to be reluctant to give mouth-to-mouth rescue breaths. To avoid the chance that the victim will not receive any care, compression-only CPR can be considered in these circumstances:

- Rescuer is unwilling or unable to perform mouth-to-mouth rescue breathing.
- Untrained bystander is following dispatcher-assisted CPR instructions.

▶ Airway Obstruction

People can choke on all kinds of objects. Foods such as candy, peanuts, and grapes are major offenders because of their shapes and consistencies. Nonfood choking deaths are often caused by balloons, balls and marbles, toys, and coins inhaled by children. Consider an athlete choking on a mouthguard, broken teeth, food, or even chewing tobacco in older athletes.

Recognizing Airway Obstruction

An object lodged in the airway can cause a mild or severe airway obstruction. In a mild airway obstruction, good air exchange is present. The victim is able to make forceful coughing efforts in an attempt to relieve the obstruction. The victim should be encouraged to cough. A victim with a severe airway obstruction will have poor air exchange. The signs of a severe airway obstruction include the following:

- Breathing becoming more difficult
- Weak and ineffective cough
- Inability to speak or breathe
- Skin, fingernail beds, and the inside of the mouth appear bluish gray (indicating cyanosis)

Choking victims sometimes clutch their necks to communicate that they are choking. This motion is known as the *universal distress signal for choking.* The victim can become panicked and desperate.

Caring for a Person with an Airway Obstruction

For a responsive adult or child with a severe airway obstruction, ask the victim "Are you choking?" If the victim is unable to respond verbally, but nods yes, provide care for the victim. Move behind the victim and reach around the victim's waist with both arms. Place a fist with the thumb side against the victim's abdomen, just above the navel. Grasp the fist with the other hand and press into the abdomen with quick inward and upward thrusts (this is the *Heimlich maneuver*). Continue thrusts until the object is removed or the victim becomes unresponsive.

If a choking victim becomes unresponsive, immediately call 9-1-1 and begin CPR. Each time the airway is opened during CPR, the rescuer should look for an object in the victim's mouth and remove it. To relieve airway obstruction in a responsive adult or child who cannot speak, breathe, or cough, follow the steps in **Skill Drill 7-3** :

1. Check the victim for choking by asking, "Are you choking?" (Step **①**).
2. Have someone call 9-1-1 or the local emergency number.
3. Take a position behind the victim and locate the victim's navel (Step **②**).
4. Place a fist with thumb side against the victim's abdomen just above the navel (Step **③**), grasp it with the other hand, and press into victim's abdomen with quick inward and upward thrusts (Step **④**). Continue thrusts until the object is removed or the victim becomes unresponsive. If the victim becomes unresponsive, call 9-1-1 and give CPR. Each time the airway is opened to give a breath, look for an object in the mouth or throat and, if seen, remove it.

skill drill

7-3 **Airway Obstruction in a Responsive Adult or Child**

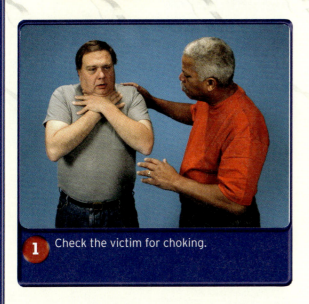

1 Check the victim for choking.

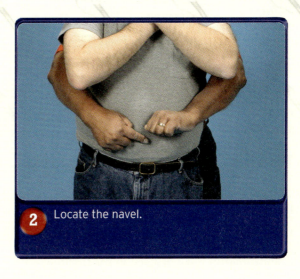

2 Locate the navel.

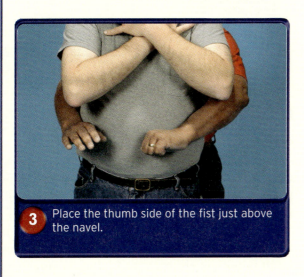

3 Place the thumb side of the fist just above the navel.

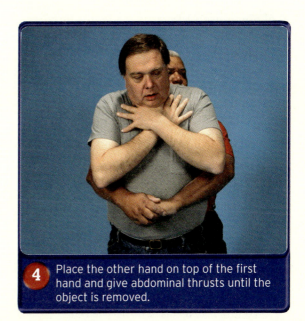

4 Place the other hand on top of the first hand and give abdominal thrusts until the object is removed.

Table 7-2 provides a review of CPR and the steps to take in the event of an airway obstruction for victims of all ages.

▶ Public Access Defibrillation

Sudden cardiac death remains an unresolved public health crisis. A victim's chances for survival are improved dramatically through early CPR and early defibrillation with the use of an AED. To be effective, defibrillation must be used in the first few minutes following cardiac arrest. The implementation of state public access defibrillation (PAD) laws and the Food and Drug Administration's (FDA) approval of home-use AEDs have made this important care step available to many rescuers in many places, including the following **Figure 7-6** :

- Airports and airplanes
- Stadiums
- Health clubs
- Golf courses
- Schools
- Government buildings
- Offices
- Homes

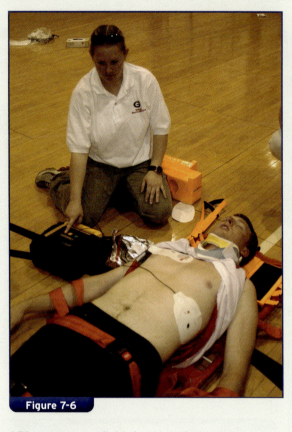

Figure 7-6

AEDs are now available in many places.

▶ About AEDs

An automated external defibrillator (AED) is an electronic device that analyzes the heart rhythm and, if necessary, delivers an electrical shock, known as *defibrillation*, to the heart of a person in cardiac arrest. The purpose of this shock is to correct one of the abnormal electrical disturbances previously discussed and to reestablish a heart rhythm that will result in normal electrical and pumping function.

All AEDs are attached to the victim by a cable connected to two adhesive pads (electrodes) placed on the victim's chest. The pad and cable system sends the electrical signal from the heart into the device for analysis and delivers the electric shock to the victim when needed **Figure 7-7** .

Table 7-2 CPR and Airway Obstruction Review

CPR
These steps are the same for all victims regardless of age:

1. Check for responsiveness and look at the chest for signs of breathing.
   - If the victim is unresponsive and has normal breathing, place the victim in the recovery position, and have someone call 9-1-1.
   - If the victim is unresponsive and has abnormal breathing (not breathing or only gasping), have someone call 9-1-1, and retrieve an AED if available. Perform Steps 2 through 5.
2. Provide chest compressions:
   - Give 30 chest compressions in the center of the victim's chest.
3. Open the airway:
   - Tilt the victim's head back and lift the chin.
4. Give 2 breaths:
   - Each breath lasts 1 second to produce visible chest rise.
5. Continue CPR until an AED is available, EMS personnel take over, or the victim starts to move.

Airway Obstruction
For responsive adults and children (anyone over age 1):

1. Check for choking.
2. Provide abdominal thrusts (Heimlich maneuver).

For responsive infants (Birth to 1 year):

1. Support the infant's head, neck and back.
2. Alternate five back blows followed by five chest compressions repeatedly.

AEDs have built-in rhythm analysis systems that determine whether the victim needs a shock. This system enables first aiders and other rescuers to deliver early defibrillation with only minimal training. AEDs also record the victim's heart rhythm (known as an *electrocardiogram,* or *ECG*), shock data, and other information about the device's performance (for example, the date, time, and number of shocks supplied) **Figure 7-8** .

Common Elements of AEDs

Many different AED models exist. The principles for use are the same for each, but the displays, controls, and options vary slightly. A coach will need to know how to use their team's specific AED. All AEDs have the following elements in common:

- Power on/off mechanism
- Cable and pads (electrodes)
- Analysis capability
- Defibrillation capability
- Prompts to guide the rescuer
- Battery operation for portability

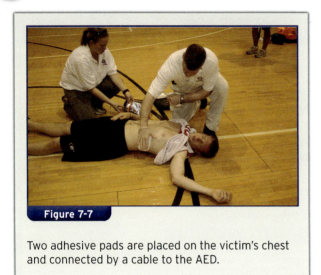

Figure 7-7

Two adhesive pads are placed on the victim's chest and connected by a cable to the AED.

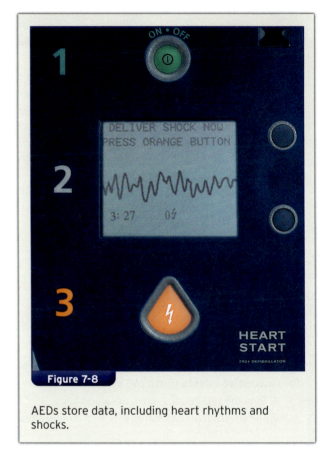

Figure 7-8

AEDs store data, including heart rhythms and shocks.

▶ Using an AED

Once EMS has been called and the need for an AED has been determined (the victim unresponsive and not breathing), the basic operation of all AED models follows this sequence `Skill Drill 7-4`:

1. Perform CPR until an AED is available (Step **❶**).
2. Once the AED is available, turn the equipment on.
3. Apply the electrode pads to the victim's bare chest and the cable to the AED (Step **❷**). If available, use child pads for a child.
4. Stand clear and analyze the heart rhythm (Step **❸**).
5. Deliver a shock if indicated.
6. Perform CPR for 2 minutes (five cycles).
7. Check the victim and repeat the analysis, shock, and CPR steps as needed (Step **❹**).

Some AEDs are powered on by pressing an on/off button. Others power on when the AED case lid is opened. Once the power is on, the AED will quickly go through some internal checks and then will begin to provide voice and screen prompts. Expose the victim's chest. The skin must be fairly dry so that the pads will adhere and conduct electricity properly. If necessary, dry the skin with a towel. Because excessive chest hair also can interfere with adhesion and electrical conduction, it may be necessary to quickly shave the area where the pads are to be placed. Razors should be kept in the case with the AED.

Remove the backing from the pads and apply them firmly to the victim's bare chest according to the diagram on the pads. One pad is placed to the right of the breastbone, just below the collarbone and above the right nipple. The second pad is placed on the left side of the chest, left of the nipple and above the lower rib margin. Make sure the cable is attached to the AED, and stand clear for an analysis of the heart's electrical activity. No one should be in contact with the victim at this time, or later if a shock is indicated.

The AED will advise if a shock is needed. Deliver the shock after verifying that no one is in contact with the victim. Begin CPR immediately following

skill drill

7-4 Using an AED

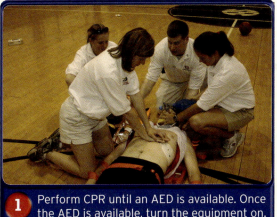

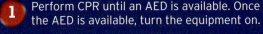

1 Perform CPR until an AED is available. Once the AED is available, turn the equipment on.

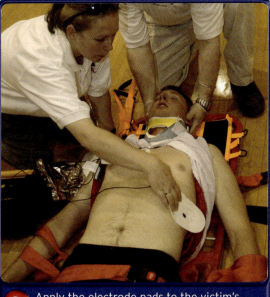

2 Apply the electrode pads to the victim's bare skin and make sure the cable is attached to the device.

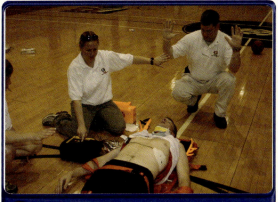

3 Stand clear and allow the device to analyze the heart rhythm. Press the shock button if advised by the device. Fully automated devices do not have a shock button and will provide the shock if needed.

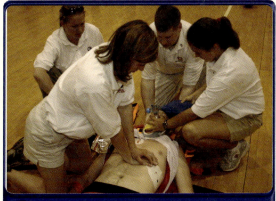

4 Perform CPR and follow the device prompts. Check the victim and repeat the analysis, shock, and CPR steps as needed.

the shock for 2 minutes (five cycles). Following CPR, recheck to see if the victim is breathing and re-analyze the rhythm. If the shock worked, the victim will begin to regain signs of life. Continue providing care until EMS personnel arrive and take over.

▶ Special Considerations

There are several special situations that a coach should be aware of when using an AED. These include water, children, medication patches, and implanted devices.

Water

Because water conducts electricity, it can provide an energy pathway between the AED and the rescuer or bystanders. Remove the victim from freestanding water. Quickly dry the chest before applying the pads. The risk to the rescuers and bystanders is very low if the chest is dry and the pads are secured to the chest.

Children

Cardiac arrest in children usually is caused by an airway or breathing problem, rather than a primary heart problem as in adults. AEDs can deliver energy levels appropriate for children age 1 month or older. If the AED has special pediatric pads and cable, use these for the child Figure 7-9 . If the pediatric equipment is not available, use an adult AED and pads.

Medication Patches

Some people wear an adhesive patch containing medication (such as nitroglycerin, nicotine, birth control, or pain medication) that is absorbed through the skin. These patches can block the delivery of energy from the pads to the heart. They need to be removed if they are located where the AED pads go; wipe the skin dry before attaching the AED pads Figure 7-10 .

Implanted Devices

Implanted pacemakers and defibrillators are small devices placed underneath the skin of people with certain types of heart disease Figure 7-11 . These devices often can be seen or felt when the chest is exposed. Avoid placing the pads directly over these devices whenever possible. If an implanted defibrillator is discharging, the victim may twitch periodically. Allow the implanted unit to stop before using the AED.

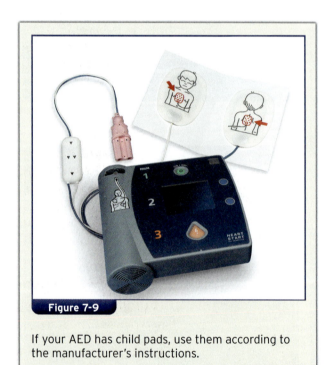

Figure 7-9

If your AED has child pads, use them according to the manufacturer's instructions.

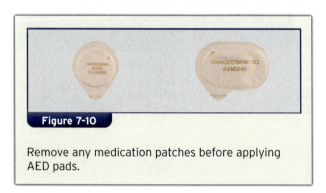

Figure 7-10

Remove any medication patches before applying AED pads.

▶ AED Maintenance

Daily inspection of the AED can ensure that the device has the necessary supplies and is in proper working condition **Figure 7-12**. AEDs conduct automatic internal checks and provide visual indications that the unit is ready and functioning properly. However, a coach does not need to turn the device on daily to check it as part of any inspection; doing so will only wear down the battery.

AED supplies should include items such as the following:

- Two sets of electrode pads with dates within the expiration period
- Extra battery
- Razor
- Hand towel
- Scissors to cut clothing

Other items to be considered are a breathing device (for example, a mask or shield) and medical exam gloves.

▶ Summary

While it is unlikely that an athlete will require CPR or use of an AED during an athletic practice or competition, it is necessary that coaches be trained in these methods of care. Proper CPR and AED use prior to EMS arrival could be the difference between life and death for the victim, whether an athlete, a coach, a referee, or a bystander.

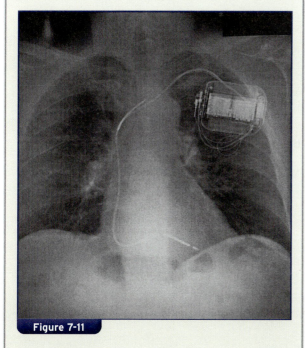

Figure 7-11

Allow an implanted defibrillator to stop before using an AED.

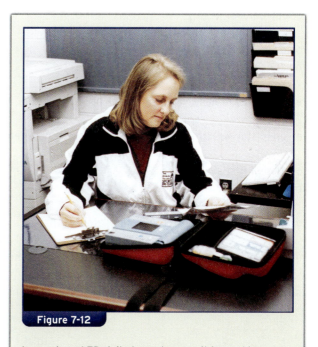

Figure 7-12

Inspect an AED daily to make sure it is working properly and has the necessary supplies.

Appendix A: Emergency Action Plan

Date: _____   Team Name: _____

Athletic Director/Team Administrator: Level of Play:
Telephone Number: Ages of Players:

On-Site Emergency Providers

Coaching Staff

Name	Level of Training

Parents

Name	Level of Training

Person who will attend to sick or injured players:
Certified in CPR and first aid?
Back-up person:

Person to call 9-1-1 in the event of an emergency:
How (phone, radio)?

Person to stay (if necessary) with a sick or injured player when the competition resumes:

Person to stay with the other players while someone attends to the sick or injured player:

Location of first-aid kit:
Contents:

Location of automated external defibrillator (AED):

Person to provide first aid if the coach is unavailable or not present:

Location of athletes' consent forms, medical history forms, and medication information:

Athletic Medical Alerts

Name	Problem

Note: *f* = figure; *t* = table

A

Abdomen
    checking, 16
    quadrants, 18*f*
Abdominal thrusts, for choking, 25
Abrasions, 32*t*
ACL (anterior cruciate ligament), 67
AEDs. *See* Automated external defibrillators
Airway assessment, 12, 14*t*, 18*f*
Airway obstruction
    care for, 92–93, 95*t*
    recognizing, 92
    tongue and, 94
Alcohol use/abuse, 9
Allergic reactions, 19*t*, 23, 25
Ambulance, 62
American football injuries, 68–69, 68*f*
Amputation, 32*t*
Anabolic steroids, 9
Anatomical splint, 37
Ankle injuries, 58, 58*t*
Anterior cruciate ligament (ACL), 67
Arm injuries
    sling for, 49
    upper, fracture of, 48, 48*f*
Assessment, 12–21
    of airway, 12, 14*t*, 18*f*
    algorithm, 13
    beginning, 11
    of breathing, 12, 14*t*, 18*f*, 87, 87*f*
    head-to-toe survey, 12, 15–17
    initial check, 12, 12*t*, 14*t*
    modifications of, 19–20, 20*t*
    responsiveness, 87, 89, 90, 91
    of responsiveness, 12, 12*t*, 14*t*, 40
    sequence for, 20*t*
Asthma, 29–30
Atherosclerosis, 86

Athletes
    female, 9
    HIV positive, 74
    injuries of (*See specific injuries*)
    injury prevention model and, 60
    judgment of, injuries and, 63
    motionless, 28–29, 29*f*
    sick/injured, approaching, 11–12
    training for, 7–8
Automated external defibrillators (AEDs)
    common elements, 95
    data storage, 95, 96*f*
    for early defibrillation, 94, 95*t*, 96, 96*f*
    maintenance, 99, 99*f*
    presence at sporting events, 28
    public access/home use, 94, 94*f*
    special considerations, 98, 98*f*
    use of, 96–98
Avulsion
    appearance/treatment of, 32*t*
    nail, 53–54

B

Back, checking, 17
Bandages
    cravat or triangular, 32
    elastic, 7
    securing dressings with, 32, 33*f*
Bandaging techniques
    for clavicle or shoulder injury, 47
    for eye injuries, 41
    for sports-related injuries, 4, 7

Barrier devices, for first-aid provider, 11
Baseball
    guidelines for number of pitches
        thrown, 8
    injuries, 74–75
Basketball injuries, 67–68
Battle's sign, 40, 40*f*
Bee stings, 31
Bites, insect, 31
Bleeding
    diagnostic algorithm, 35
    from wounds, 32–34, 32*t*, 33*f*
Blisters, 34, 34*f*
Blood glucose, low, 25
Blunt trauma, to chest, 44
Brain injury
    assessing level of responsiveness, 40
    care for, 39–40
    diagnosis, 39
Breathing
    abnormal sounds, 14*t*
    absence of, 28–29, 29*f*
    assessment of, 12, 14*t*, 18*f*, 87, 87*f*
    problems, 29–30, 85*t*
Bruises. *See* Contusions
Buddy splint
    finger, 53, 53*f*
    leg, 55, 55*f*
Burns, 34, 36

C

CABD mnemonic, 12, 14*t*
Cardiac arrest
    in baseball/softball players, 74
    care for, 87, 87*f*
    prevalence, 84–85
Cardiac contusions, 44–45, 85*t*
Cardiac problems. *See* Heart problems

Chain of survival, 85–86, 86*f*
Cheerleading injuries, 76
Chemical burns, 34, 36
Chest
    checking, 16
    compressions, 84, 88–91
    injuries, 44–45, 45*f*
Children
    automated external defibrillators and,
        98, 98*f*
    CPR for, 89, 91
Choking
    care for, 25, 25*f*
    signs/symptoms, 92
    universal distress signal for, 25,
        25*f*, 92
Circulation, 19
Clavicle fracture, 46, 47
Cleaning, of contaminated area, 12
Clothing, improvised slings from,
    48, 50*f*
Coaches
    anticipation of potential injuries, 3
    injury of, 11
    injury prevention (*See* Injury
        prevention)
    injury prevention model and, 61
    liability minimization, 3–4
    minimizing risk, 3–4
    postinjury phase and, 63–64
    protection of, 11
    return-to-play decision making, 2–3,
        21–22
    suspicion of player illness/injury,
        10–11
    training, reasons for, 2–3
Cold-related emergencies, 26
Cold therapy, 7
Collarbone, 46
Collateral ligament injuries, 56

Commotio cordis, 44, 74, 85*t*

Compression, in RICE mnemonic, 4, 6

Compression only CPR, 92

Concussions
  brain injuries and, 39–40
  definition of, 8
  multiple, 8
  symptoms, 40

Conditioning, 7–8, 60, 75

Confidentiality, 4

Consent forms, 4

Contact/collision sports
  basketball, 67–68
  football, 68–69, 68*f*
  ice hockey, 69–70, 69*f*
  listing of, 66*t*

Contusions (bruises)
  brain injuries and, 39
  cardiac, 44–45, 85*t*
  care for, 36
  causes of, 36
  fibula, 57
  muscle, 55–56
  shoulder, 46
  tibia, 57

Coronary arteries, 86

CPR
  adult, 89, 90
  breathing check, 87, 87*f*
  chest compressions, 88–91
  child, 89, 91
  compression only, 92
  early, 86
  rescue breaths, 87–88, 88*f*
  responsiveness check, 87
  steps in, 14*t*, 95*t*

Cravat (triangular bandage), 32

Crepitus, 37

Cruciate ligament injuries, 56

D

Decision to return to play, 21–22

Defibrillation. *See also* Automated external
      defibrilators
  definition of, 94
  early, 86
  public access, 94, 94*f*

Deformity, 12, 37

Diabetic emergencies, 25

Diaphragm spasm, 30

Diet, 66–67

Disease transmission, 11

Dislocations
  care for, 36
  definition of, 36
  finger, 53
  hip, 54–55, 55*f*
  knee, 56
  kneecap, 56
  shoulder, 46

Doctor's clearance, 40

Doctor visit, situations requiring, 21

Documentation, 4

DOTS exam, 12, 15–17, 37

Dressings
  for chest injuries, 45
  for wound care, 32, 33*f*

Drinking, while providing care, 12

Drowning, 36–37

Drug use/abuse
  anabolic steroids, 9
  causing heart problems, 85*t*
  overdose/poisoning from, 25–26

Duty of care, 4

E

EAP (emergency action plan), 11, 61–62, 100

Ears, checking, 15

Eating, while providing care, 12
ECG (electrocardiogram), 95–96
Elbow
    fractures/dislocations, 48, 51, 51*f*
    tennis elbow, 51
Electrical burns, 34, 36
Electrical defibrillation, 84
Electrocardiogram (ECG), 95–96
Electrolyte-containing fluids, 8
Elevation, in RICE mnemonic, 4, 6
Emergency action plan (EAP), 11,
        61–62, 100
Emergency medical services (EMS)
    activation, 12, 14*t*, 95*t*
    information for dispatcher,
        20–21
Environment, preinjury phase and, 61
Environmental emergencies
    cold-related, 26
    heat-related, 27
Equipment, malfunction, 63
Events, leading to injury/illness, 19*t*
Extremities, checking, 17
Eye/eyes
    injuries, 41
    protection, for first-aid provider, 11
    "raccoon eyes," 40, 40*f*

F

Facial injuries, 41–42
Fainting/faintness, 27
Female athletes, 9
Femur fractures, 55
Fibula
    contusion, 57
    fracture, 56–57, 57*f*
Field event injuries, 77–78, 77*f*

Finger/fingers
    dislocation, 11, 53
    fracture, 52–53, 53*f*
    sprained or jammed, 53
First aid
    definition of, 3
    general principles, 4, 6–7
    law and, 3–4
    risks from providing, 11
First-aid providers, protection of, 11
Football injuries, 68–69, 68*f*
Fractures
    applying splint, 37–38, 38*f*
    care of, 37
    clavicle, 46, 47
    femur, 55
    fibula, 56–57, 57*f*
    finger, 52–53, 53*f*
    hip, 55
    knee, 56
    radius, 52
    recognition of, 37
    skull, 40–41, 40*f*
    spinal, 43
    tibia, 56–57, 57*f*
    tooth, 42
    ulna, 52
    upper arm, 48, 48*f*
    vs. sprains, 38
    wrist, 52, 53*f*
Frostbite, 26

G

Gasping respirations, 14*t*
Gender differences, 9
Gloves, for first-aid provider, 11
Golfer's elbow, 51–52

Gurgling breath, 14*t*
Gymnastics, 77–78

H

Hamstring injuries, 60
Head injuries, 39–42, 39*f*
Head tilt–chin lift, 90
Head-to-toe survey, 12, 15–19
Heart
    anatomy, 86, 86*f*
    physiology of, 86, 86*f*
Heart problems
    cardiac arrest (*See* Cardiac arrest)
    cardiac contusions, 44–45, 85*t*
    causes of, 84–85, 85*t*
    commotio cordis, 44, 74, 85*t*
    heart attack, 28, 84–85
    underlying, 85*t*
Heat cramps, 27
Heat exhaustion, 27
Heat stroke, 27
Heat therapy, 7
Heimlich maneuver, 25, 95*t*
Helmets
    HECC certification standards, 69
    lacrosse, 70
    proper fit, 68, 68*f*
    removal guidelines for, 42
Help seeking, 4, 20–21
Hematoma, 39
Hepatitis B, 11
Hip
    dislocation, 54–55, 55*f*
    fracture, 55
HIV-positive athletes, 74
Homemade ice packs, 7
Hospital visit, situations requiring, 21

Hydration, 8
Hyperventilation Syndrome, 28
Hypothermia, 26

I

Ice, in RICE mnemonic, 4, 6
Ice hockey injuries, 69–70, 69*f*
Ice massage, 7
Ice packs
    homemade, 7
    precautions, 7
Illness. *See also specific illnesses*
    approaching a sick athlete, 11–12
    recognition of, 10–11
    sudden, diagnostic algorithm for, 24
Immunization status, of coach, 11, 12
ImPACT (Immediate Post-Concussion Assessment and Cognitive Test), 8
Implanted devices, automated external defibrillators and, 98, 99*f*
Incisions, 32*t*
Infections, wound, 34
Infectious disease, transmission of, 11
Initial check, 12, 12*t*, 14*t*
Initial response algorithm, 13
Injuries. *See also specific injuries*
    approaching an injured athlete, 11–12
    recognition of, 10–11
    severity of, 21
Injury phase, of injury prevention model, 62–63
Injury prevention
    alpine skiing, 78
    baseball/softball, 75
    basketball, 67–68
    cheerleading, 76
    field events, 77

Injury prevention (*cont.*)
  football, 68–69, 68*f*
  gymnastics, 78
  ice hockey, 69–70, 69*f*
  lacrosse, 70–71
  martial arts, 71
  roller hockey, 72
  soccer, 72–73, 73*f*
  strategies for, 3
  swimming, 79–80, 80*f*
  tennis, 80–81
  track, 81, 81*f*
  volleyball, 79
  weight lifting/weight training, 81–83,
    82–83, 82*f*
  wrestling, 73–74, 74*f*
Injury prevention model, 59–64, 60*f*
  injury phase, 62–63
  postinjury phase, 63–64
  preinjury phase, 60–62, 62*f*
  purpose of, 59–60
Inline hockey injuries, 71–72
Insect bites/stings, 31

J

Jammed finger, 53
Joint dislocations, 36
Judo injuries, 71

K

Karate injuries, 71
Knee
  dislocation, 56
  fractures, 56
  sprain, 56
Kneecap dislocation, 56

L

Lacerations, 32*t*
Lacrosse injuries, 70–71
LAF exam, 12, 15–17
Leg, lower, fractures of, 56–57, 57*f*
Limited contact sports
  alpine skiing, 78
  baseball/softball, 74–75
  cheerleading, 75–76
  field events, 77–78, 77*f*
  listing of, 66*t*
Little league elbow, 51–52
Lower extremity
  anatomy, 54*f*
  injuries, 54–58, 55*f*, 57*f*, 58*t*
    (*See also specific lower
    extremity injuries*)

M

Manual spinal stabilization, 44, 44*f*
Martial arts injuries, 71
Medical care, additional, recommendations
    for, 21
Medical clearance, 22
Medical problems, pertinent, 19*t*
Medical team, injury prevention model and,
    61–62
Medical waste, 11
Medication patches, automated external
    defibrillators and, 98, 98*f*
Medications. *See also* Drug use/abuse
  ingestion, causing heart
    problems, 85*t*
  labeling, 61, 62*f*
  overdose/poisoning from, 25–26
  in SAMPLE history, 19*t*
Memory loss, short-term, 40

Mental state alterations
    concussions and, 8
    in diabetic emergency, 25
Motionless athlete, 28–29, 29*f*
Mouth
    checking, 15
    injuries, 41–42
Mouth-to-barrier device, 88, 88*f*
Mouth-to-nose method, of rescue
        breathing, 88
Mouth-to-stoma method, of rescue
        breathing, 88–89
Movement, checking, 19
Muscle contusions, 55–56
Muscle cramps/spasms, 57

N

Nail
    avulsion, 53–54
    blood under, 54
Neck, checking, 15
Negligence, 4
9-1-1 phone calls, 12, 14*t*, 20
Noncontact sports
    listing of, 66*t*
    swimming, 79–80, 80*f*
    tennis, 80–81
Nose
    checking, 15
    injuries, 42

O

Officials, injury prevention model and, 61
Open wounds, 12, 37
Oral intake, last, 19*t*
Ottawa Ankle Rules, 58, 58*t*

P

PAD (public access defibrillation), 94, 94*f*
Pain, 37
Patella dislocation, 56
Pelvis, checking, 17
Performance-enhancing drugs, 9
Performance-enhancing hydrating fluids, 8
Petit mal seizures, 29
Pillow splint, 57, 57*f*
Poisoning, 25–26
Positioning, of victim, 14*t*, 88
Postinjury phase, 63–64
Power volleyball injuries, 78–79
Preinjury phase, 60
Protective equipment. *See under specific*
        sports
Public access defibrillation (PAD), 94, 94*f*
Pulse taking, 19
Puncture wounds, 32*t*
Pupils, checking, 15

R

Raccoon eyes, 40, 40*f*
Radius fracture, 52
Range-of-motion (ROM) testing, 19
Raynaud's disease, 7
Record keeping, 3
Repetitive stress/overuse injuries, 8
Reporting of illness/injury, 4
Rescue breathing, 87–91, 88*f*
Responsiveness checking. *See also*
        Unresponsiveness
    CPR and, 87, 89, 90, 91
    methods for, 12, 12*t*, 40
Rest, in RICE mnemonic, 4, 6
Return-to-play decision, 10, 21–22
Return-to-play note, 21

RICE, 4, 6
Roller hockey injuries, 71–72
ROM testing (range-of-motion testing), 19
Rules of the game, injury prevention model
        and, 61

S

SAMPLE history, 19, 19*t*
SAM splint, 37
SA node (sinoatrial node), 86*f*
Scalp wounds, 41
Scapula, 46
Second-impact syndrome, 40
Seizures, 29
Sensation, checking, 19
Shin splints, 57–58
Shortness of breath, 29–30
Short-term memory loss, 40
Shoulder injuries
        bandaging, 47
        contusions, 46
        dislocations, 46
        tendinitis, 48
Shoulder pointers, 46
Sickness. *See* Illness
Sinoatrial node (SA node), 86*f*
Skiing (alpine), 78
Skin
        color, 15
        moisture, 18*t*
        temperature, 15, 18*t*
Skull fracture, 40–41, 40*f*
Slings
        for arm injury, 49
        improvised, 48, 50*f*
        sling and swathe method, 37, 38*f*, 47
Snoring, 14*t*
Soccer injuries, 72–73, 73*f*

Softball injuries, 74–75
Spinal column, anatomy, 43*f*
Spinal cord injuries, 43–44
        effect on victim's life, 9
        manual stabilization, 44, 44*f*
        prevalence, 9
        stabilization for, 15
        symptoms, 17
Splinters, 54
Splints
        application methods, 37–38, 38*f*
        buddy, 53, 53*f*, 55, 55*f*
        materials for, 38
        pillow, 57, 57*f*
        rigid, 52, 53*f*
Sports
        classification by contact, 65–66, 66*t*
                (*See also specific sports*)
Sports first aid. *See* First aid
Sports first-aid kit, contents of,
        4, 5*t*
Sprains
        care for, 38
        definition of, 38
        finger, 53
        knee, 56
        vs. fractures, 38
        vs. strains, 39
Stabilization, manual spinal, 44, 44*f*
Steri-strips, 33
Stings, insect, 31
Stoma, 89
Stomach distention, 88
Strains, 39
Stridor, 14*t*
Sunburn, 36
Sunscreen, 73*f*
Suturing, of wounds, 33–34
Swelling, 12, 37
Swimming injuries, 79–80, 80*f*

Symptoms. *See also under specific injuries*
requiring immediate care, 20
SAMPLE history and, 19t

Upper extremity injuries, 45–54, 45f, 48f,
50f, 51f, 53f. (*See also specific upper
extremity injuries*)

T

Tackle football injuries, 68–69, 68f
Tae Kwon Do injuries, 71
Teeth
fractured, 42
knocked-out, 42
Tenderness, 12, 37
Tendinitis, shoulder area, 48
Tennis elbow, 51
Tennis injuries, 80–81
Tetanus, 11
Thermal burns, 34, 36
Thighbone (femur), 55
Thigh injuries, 55
Tibia
contusion, 57
fracture, 56–57, 57f
Toe injuries, 58
Tongue, airway obstruction and, 94
Track injuries, 81, 81f
Training, 7–8

U

Ulna fracture, 52
Underhydration, 8
Universal distress signal for choking, 25,
25f, 92
Unresponsiveness
care for, 30
in diabetic emergency, 25
spinal injuries and, 43

V

Ventricular fibrillation (V-fib), 87
Ventricular tachycardia (V-tach), 87
Victim assessment. *See* Assessment
Volleyball injuries, 78–79
Vomiting, 30

W

Waste disposal containers, 11
Water
AEDs and, 98
hydration and, 8
Water bottles, sharing, 8
Weight lifting/weight training injuries,
81–83, 82f
Weight loss, for wrestling, 74
Wheezing, 14t
Wounds
bleeding from, 32–34, 32t, 33f
care for, 32–34
diagnostic algorithm, 35
dressings for, 11
infected, 34
open, 12, 37
suturing, 33–34
Wrestling injuries, 73–74, 74f

Y

Youth sports coaches. *See* Coaches

image credits

Chapter 1
Opener © KennStilger47/ShutterStock, Inc.

Chapter 2
Opener © Sergey I/ShutterStock, Inc.

Chapter 3
3-1 Courtesy of Anatoly Myaskovsky.

Chapter 4
4-1, 4-2, 4-3, 4-7 Courtesy of Nicholas Palmieri;
4.12a Photographed by Kimberly Potvin

Chapter 5
Opener © iofoto/ShutterStock, Inc.; 5-2 Photographed by
Christine McKeen.

Chapter 6
Opener © Alan C. Heison/ShutterStock, Inc.; 6-1 ©
Stephen Coburn/ShutterStock, Inc.; 6-2 © Amy Myers/
ShutterStock, Inc.; 6-3 Courtesy of Nicholas Palmieri;
6-4 Photographed by Christine McKeen; 6-5 © Larry St.
Pierre/ShutterStock, Inc.; 6-6 © Dennis MacDonald/Alamy
Images; 6-7 © Photos.com; 6-8 © Johann Helgason/
ShutterStock, Inc.; 6-9 © VLDR/ShutterStock, Inc.

Chapter 7
7-1 Source: American Heart Association; 7-8, 7-9 Philips
HeartStart FR2+ Defibrillator, used with permission of
Philips Healthcare. All rights reserved.

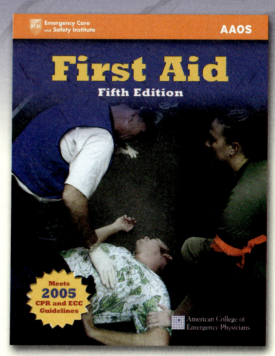
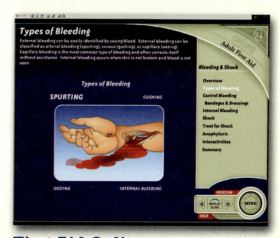

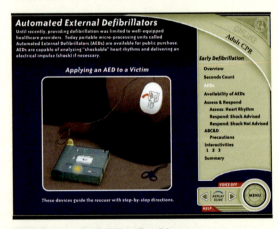

Additional Resources from the Emergency Care and Safety Institute

ECSI offers dynamic, Flash™-based safety and emergency response courses online that will teach you how to prevent injuries and illnesses, as well as what to do if an emergency occurs.

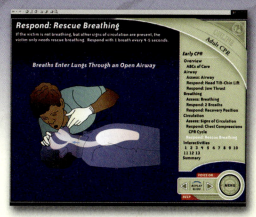

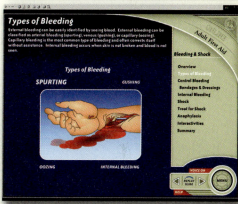

Distance learning enables students and instructors to work either independently or together. Students can review course content anytime, at any place, making learning both easy and convenient. ECSI's online courses can stand alone, be used in conjunction with traditional classroom-based courses, or be used as "blended training" with separate skill labs/assessments provided after completion of the knowledge portion of the course online. ECSI offers the flexibility of mixing distance learning courses with physical, on-site activities.

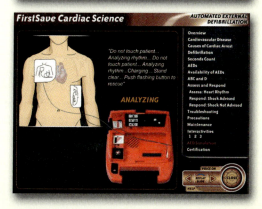

To preview any of ECSI's online courses, call 1-800-832-0034 or visit www.ECSInstitute.org today.

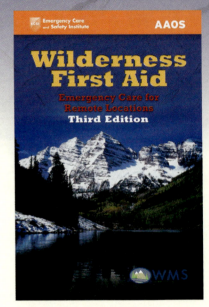
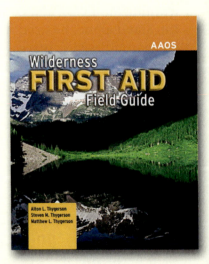

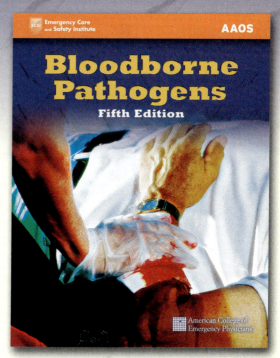
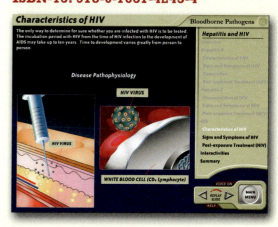

Interactive courses to help you prepare for caring for infants and children.

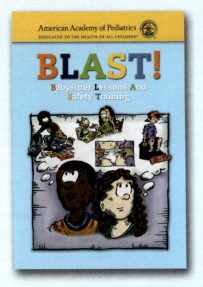

An interactive version of BLAST! is also available on CD-ROM.
Use ISBN-13: 978-0-7637-3517-3

Babysitter Lessons and Safety Training (BLAST!)
American Academy of Pediatrics
ISBN-13: 978-0-7637-3516-6

BLAST! is an important training program for potential babysitters and parents considering hiring a babysitter. Brought to you by the American Academy of Pediatrics, **BLAST!** is exciting and interactive, providing extensive training in pediatric first aid, household safety, and the fundamentals of childcare.

BLAST! features babysitter basics including:
- Feeding
- Burping
- Spoon-feeding
- Managing crying
- Preparing for bed
- Behavioral problems
- Discipline
- An introduction to first aid

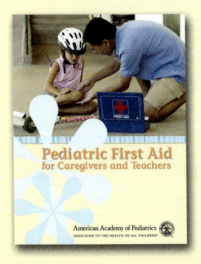

Pediatric First Aid for Caregivers and Teachers (PedFACTS), Revised First Edition
American Academy of Pediatrics
ISBN-13: 978-0-7637-4404-5

PedFACTs is a national pediatric first aid course instructing caregivers and teachers in what they need to know when a child is injured or becomes suddenly and severely ill. Most injuries that require first aid are not life-threatening. Usually, first aid involves simple, common sense procedures. However, first aid can sometimes mean the difference between life and death. All caregivers and teachers should have pediatric first aid training!

Visit **www.PedFACTSonline.com** to learn more today!

Notes

Notes

Notes

Notes